THE PEDIATRIC BOOK OF LISTS

A Primer of Differential Diagnosis in

Pediatrics

THE PEDIATRIC BOOK OF LISTS
A Primer of Differential Diagnosis in Pediatrics

JAMES A. STOCKMAN III, M.D.

Professor and Chairman of Pediatrics
Associate Dean, Northwestern University
  Medical School
Centennial Chairman of Medicine and
  Physician-in-Chief
The Children's Memorial Hospital
Chicago, Illinois

TIMOTHY E. CORDEN, M.D.

Instructor in Pediatrics
Northwestern University Medical School
Chief Resident Physician in Pediatrics
The Children's Memorial Hospital
Chicago, Illinois

JULIE J. KIM, M.D.

Instructor in Pediatrics
Northwestern University Medical School
Chief Resident Physician in Pediatrics
The Children's Memorial Hospital
Chicago, Illinois

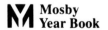
Mosby
Year Book

St. Louis   Baltimore   Boston   Chicago   London   Philadelphia   Sydney   Toronto

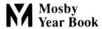
Mosby Year Book

Dedicated to Publishing Excellence

Sponsoring Editor: James F. Shanahan
Associate Managing Editor, Manuscript Services: Deborah Thorp
Production Coordinator: Nancy Baker
Proofroom Supervisor: Barbara Kelly

Mosby-Year Book, Inc.
11830 Westline Industrial Drive
St. Louis, MO 63146

1 2 3 4 5 6 7 8 9 0 CL/MA 95 94 93 92 91

Library of Congress Cataloging-in-Publication Data
Stockman, James A., 1943-
    The pediatric book of lists: a primer of differential diagnosis in pediatrics / James A. Stockman III, Timothy E. Corden, Julie J. Kim.
        p.   cm.
    Includes bibliographical references.
    Includes index.
    ISBN 0-8151-8321-6
    1. Diagnosis, Differential. 2. Pediatrics. I. Corden, Timothy E. II. Kim, Julie J. III. Title.
    [DNLM: 1. Diagnosis, Differential—in infancy & childhood—handbooks. WS 39 S865p]
    RJ51.D53S76 1991
    618.92'0075—dc20   91-13512
    DNLM/DLC   CIP
    for Library of Congress

To the Residents in Pediatrics, Graduate Training
Program, Northwestern University Medical School and The
Children's Memorial Hospital for their dedication both
to patient care and to the pursuit of medical
knowledge.

PREFACE

To all the wise and the otherwise

This book is indeed intended for everyone. We have written this to provide a means of having handy the most useful of pediatric facts. What puzzles us most often is determining the cause of what we observe. The solution to the puzzle is the "differential diagnosis." This book contains over 350 lists, selected from among the most frequently asked questions on rounds and during morning reports. Obviously, this work is not intended to be comprehensive and, certainly, is not a substitute for standard textbooks of Pediatrics. The authors would appreciate hearing from you and learning what other "tables" of facts you have found helpful in your daily activities. We will gladly acknowledge them.

Several individuals have made important contributions to this book. The residents of Children's Memorial Hospital, especially, Jennifer Myhre, Barry Ticho, Christina Rodriquez, and Linda Rufer, indeed made this work possible. We are especially grateful to our prize secretary, Linda Groble, for the preparation of the manuscript.

James A. Stockman III, M.D.
Timothy E. Corden, M.D.
Julie J. Kim, M.D.

CONTENTS

CHAPTER I

ALLERGY

COMMON DISEASES IN THE DIFFERENTIAL DIAGNOSIS OF ASTHMA

FOREIGN BODY ASPIRATION
CYSTIC FIBROSIS
CONGENITAL VASCULAR MALFORMATION
CONGENITAL TRACHEAL MALFORMATION
LARYNGOTRACHEAL MALACIA
GASTROESOPHAGEAL REFLUX
BRONCHIOLITIS OBLITERANS (RSV,
  ADENOVIRUS)
SINUSITIS
IMMOTILE CILIA SYNDROME
RIGHT MIDDLE LOBE SYNDROME

Modified from: *Principles and Practice of Pediatrics*, Oski FA, DeAngelis CD, Feigin RD, Warshaw JB (eds), J.B. Lippincott, Philadelphia, 1990, p.206.

WEATHER CHANGES REPORTED TO PRECIPITATE ASTHMATIC ATTACKS

DECREASE IN TEMPERATURE
DECREASE IN HUMIDITY
INCREASE IN HUMIDITY
DECREASE IN BAROMETRIC PRESSURE
INCREASE IN BAROMETRIC PRESSURE
DECREASE IN WIND VELOCITY

Modified from: *Pediatric Allergy*, Sly MR (ed), Medical Examination Publishing Co, Inc., New Hyde Park, 1985, p.53.

HIGH RISK FACTORS OF ASTHMATIC CHILDREN HOSPITALIZED AT THE NATIONAL JEWISH CENTER FOR IMMUNOLOGY AND RESPIRATORY MEDICINE

SEIZURES WITH ASTHMA
POOR SELF CARE
DENIAL OF WHEEZING
DEPRESSION
PARENT AND STAFF CONFLICT
PREDNISONE REDUCTION OF GREATER THAN 50%
  OF THE INITIAL DOSE
INCREASED WHEEZING THE WEEK PRIOR TO
  DISCHARGE

ASSOCIATED FACTORS
  Emotional disturbance
  History of emotional, behavioral, and
    physical reactions to separation or
    loss
  Manipulative use of asthma within the
    family
  Family dysfunction
  Patient and staff conflict
  Patient and parent conflict
  Use of inhaled beclomethasone at
    hospital discharge

Modified from: *Allergic Diseases from Infancy to
Adulthood*, Bierman CW, Pearlman DS (eds), 2nd Edition,
W.B. Saunders Company, Philadelphia, 1988, p.609.

FACTORS AFFECTING THEOPHYLLINE CLEARANCE

  INCREASED CLEARANCE
    Cigarette smoking
    Phenytoin
    Charcoal broiled meats
    High protein diet
    Phenobarbital
    Isoproterenol
  DECREASED CLEARANCE
    Prematurity
    Newborn
    Cirrhosis
    Congestive heart failure
    Fever
    Acute viral illness
    Cimetidine
    Erythromycin
    Renal failure
    Dietary xanthines
    High carbohydrate diet
    Troleandomycin
    Allopurinol
    Propranolol
    Influenza vaccine
    Oral contraceptives

Modified from: *Principles and Practice of Pediatrics*,
Oski FA, DeAngelis CD, Feigin RD, Warshaw JB (eds), J.B.
Lippincott, Philadelphia, 1990, p.203.

Pediatric Allergy, Sly MR (ed), Medical Examination
Publishing Company, Inc., 1985, p.111

ADVERSE EFFECTS OF PARENTAL SMOKING ON THEIR OFFSPRING

PREPARTUM
Increased still births
Increased neonatal death rates
Increased abortions (?)
Lowered average birthweights
Increased cord IgE

POSTPARTUM
Increased persistent wheezing (up to fourfold)
Increased serous otitis media (twofold)
Increased serum IgE (twofold)
Earlier onset of respiratory allergies
Increased specific IgE to pollen and foods

Modified from: *Allergy Principles and Practice*, Middleton E Jr, Reed CE, Ellis EF, Adkinson NF, Yuninger JW (eds), 3rd Edition, C.V. Mosby Company, St. Louis, 1988, p.947.

COMPLICATIONS OF CORTICOSTEROID THERAPY

ENDOCRINE
Diabetes mellitus
Delayed sexual maturation
Secondary amenorrhea
Adrenal insufficiency

METABOLIC
Hyperlipidemia
Hypokalemia
Sodium retention
Centripetal obesity
Negative nitrogen balance

MUSCULOSKELETAL
Growth retardation (decreased somatomedin)
Osteoporosis
Myopathy
Aseptic necrosis of bone

IMMUNOLOGIC
Leukocyte redistribution
Impaired macrophage function
Impaired inflammatory response
Increased susceptibility to infection

OTHER
>Peptic ulcer
>Pancreatitis
>Glaucoma
>Posterior subcapsular cataracts
>Psychosis
>Pseudotumor cerebri
>Hypertension
>Subcutaneous tissue atrophy
>Impaired wound healing

Modified from: *Allergic Diseases from Infancy to Adulthood*, Bierman CW, Pearlman DS (eds), 2nd Edition, W.B. Saunders Company, Philadelphia, 1988, p.205.

CONDITIONS PREDISPOSING OR ASSOCIATED WITH CHRONIC SINUSITIS IN CHILDHOOD

LOCAL FACTORS
>Nasal obstruction
>>Choanal atresia
>>Septal deviations
>>Foreign bodies
>>Polyps
>>Hypertrophied adenoids (infected?)
>>Tumors
>>Trauma
>>Swimming
>>Rhinitis medicamentosa
>>Teeth infections

SYSTEMIC DISEASES
>Viral upper respiratory tract infections
>Allergic
>>Rhinitis
>>Asthma
>Cystic fibrosis
>Immune disorders
>Immotile cilia syndrome
>Down syndrome
>Idiosyncratic reactions to aspirin and other drugs

Modified from: Rachelefsky GS, Katz RM, Siegel SC: *Pediatric Clinics of North America* 35:1043, 1988.

RISK FACTORS IN DEVELOPMENT OF ATOPY

    HEREDITY (PARENTAL ATOPY)
    INCREASED ALLERGEN EXPOSURE
        Brief breast feeding
        Allergens in breast milk
        Early solid food feeding
        Increased household mite and pet
          exposure
        Month or season of birth or weaning
    SPECIFIC VIRAL INFECTIONS
    EXPOSURE TO EXCESSIVE CIGARETTE SMOKE
    SPECIFIC INFANT IMMUNOLOGIC
      CHARACTERISTICS
        Increased cord or serum IgE
        Increased specific IgE (egg, mite)
        Decreased T (T_8 subset) cells
        Increased peripheral eosinophilia
        Increased nasal eosinophilia/
          basophilia
        Increased monocyte C-AMP
          phosphodiesterase activity
    CLINICAL SIGNS
        Recurrent wheezing in infancy
        Recurrent croup

Modified from: *Allergy Principles and Practice*,
Middleton E Jr, Reed CE, Ellis EF, Adkinson NF,
Yunginger JW (eds), 3rd Edition, C.V. Mosby Company,
St. Louis, 1988, p.961.

MAJOR CAUSES OF URTICARIA AND ANGIOEDEMA

    DRUG REACTIONS
    FOODS
    INFECTION
    INHALANTS
    INSECTS
    SYSTEMIC DISEASES
        Collagen vascular diseases
        Malignancy
        Endocrine disorders
    URTICARIA PIGMENTOSA AND SYSTEMIC
      MASTOCYTOSIS

HEREDITARY DISORDERS
    Familial cold urticaria
    Hereditary vibratory angioedema
    Urticaria with amyloidosis, deafness,
        and limb pain
    Hereditary angioedema (HAE)
PHYSICAL URTICARIAS
    Dermatographism
    Cholinergic urticaria
    Exercise-induced anaphylactic syndrome
    Familial and acquired cold urticaria
    Localized and acquired cold urticaria
    Aquagenic urticaria
    Delayed pressure urticaria/angioedema
    Solar urticaria
    Familial and acquired vibratory
        angioedema
CHRONIC IDIOPATHIC DISORDERS

Modified from: *Principles and Practice of Pediatrics*,
Oski FA, DeAngelis CD, Feigin RD, Warshaw JB (eds), J.B.
Lippincott, Philadelphia, 1990, p.209.

PARTIAL LIST OF FOODS AND BEVERAGES
LIKELY TO CONTAIN SULFITES

BEER AND WINE
CITRUS DRINKS
SHRIMP AND OTHER SEAFOODS
POTATOES - BAKED, FRIED, CHIPS, SALAD
FRESH AND DRIED FRUITS AND VEGETABLES
PREPARED VEGETABLES (CELLOPHANE PACKAGES)
SALADS
CIDER AND VINEGAR
AVOCADOS AND GUACAMOLE
FRESH RED MEAT
READY-MADE FOODS

Modified from: *Allergy Principles and Practice*,
Middleton E Jr, Reed CE, Ellis EF, Adkinson NF, Yunginger JW
(eds), 3rd Edition, C.V. Mosby Company, St. Louis, 1988,
p.1556.

COMMON CAUSES OF ANAPHYLAXIS

IgE-MEDIATED AGENTS
- Antibiotics
    - Penicillins
    - Cephalosporins
    - Tetracyclines
    - Nitrofurantoin
    - Streptomycin
    - Vancomycin
    - Chloramphenicol
    - Bacitracin
    - Neomycin
    - Polymyxin B (?)*
    - Kanamycin
    - Amphotericin B
- Foreign protein agents
    - Heterologous serum
    - ACTH
    - Insulin
    - Parathyroid hormone
    - Asparaginase
    - Chymotrypsin
    - Trypsin
    - Penicillinase
    - Relexin
    - Seminal plasma
    - Hymenoptera venom
    - Kissing bug saliva (Triatoma)
    - Vasopressin
    - Antilymphocyte globulin
    - Deerfly venom
    - Rattlesnake venom
    - Acasia
    - Glue
    - Protamine
    - Fire ant venom
    - Jellyfish protein
- Therapeutic agents
    - Allergen extracts
    - Muscle relaxants (some reactions)
    - Estradiol
    - Hydrocortisone
    - Methylprednisolone
    - Benzylpenicilloylpolylysine (Pre-pen)
    - Procaine (?)*
    - Tripelennamine
    - Ethylene oxide gas
    - Thiopental

                    Local anesthetics (some reactions)
                    Mannitol (?)*
                    Vaccines
                    Streptokinase
                    Ethylene oxide
            Foods
                    Milk
                    Egg white
                    Shellfish
                    Legumes
                    Nuts
                    Citrus fruits
                            Bananas
                            Grains
                            Sunflower seeds
                            Chocolate
                            Fish
                            Beets
                            Mango
                            Cottonseed
                            Corn
                            Safflower
                            Chamomile tea
                            Metabisulfites
    IMMUNE COMPLEX- OR COMPLEMENT-MEDIATED
      AGENTS
            Whole blood
            Cryoprecipitate
            Immunoglobulin
            Plasma
            Radiocontrast media (?)*
            Methotrexate
    MODULATORS OF ARACHIDONIC ACID
      METABOLISM
            Acetylsalicylic acid
            Nonsteroidal anti-inflammatory
              agents
            Benzoates (presumed)
            Tartrazine (possibly)
    DIRECT HISTAMINE-RELEASING AGENTS
            Opiates
            Curare, ditubocurarine
            Radiocontrast media
            Sodium dehydracholate (?)*
            Sulfobromophthalein (BSP) (?)*
            Dextran

*   Precise mechanism not established; this is a
    presumptive classification.

Iron-dextran (?)*
Thiamine (?)*
Mannitol
Pentamidine
Many chemotherapeutic agents
Polymixin B

*   Precise mechanism not established; this
is a presumptive classification.

Modified from: *Allergy Principles and Practice*,
Middleton E Jr, Reed CE, Ellis EF, Adkinson NF,
Yuninger JW (eds), 3rd Edition, C.V. Mosby Company,
St. Louis, 1988, pp.1366-1367.

HYMENOPTERA THAT MOST FREQUENTLY CAUSE ANAPHYLACTIC REACTIONS

HONEYBEE
BUMBLEBEE
YELLOW JACKET
PAPER WASP
WHITE FACED HORNET
FIRE ANT

Modified from: *Pediatric Allergy*, Sly MR (ed),
Medical Examination Publishing Company, Inc., New Hyde
Park, 1985, p.283.

PROPOSED MECHANISMS FOR BENEFIT FROM IMMUNOTHERAPY

INCREASED IgG BLOCKING ANTIBODY
INCREASED SECRETORY IgA ANTIBODY
BLUNTED IgE ANTIBODY RESPONSE TO
   INHALANT ALLERGENS
DECREASED LYMPHOCYTE RESPONSE
DECREASED BASOPHIL SENSITIVITY
DECREASED LATE-PHASE REACTION

Modified from: Eggleston PA: *Pediatric Clinics of
North America* 35:1107, 1988.

NONSTEROIDAL ANTI-INFLAMMATORY DRUGS THAT CROSS-REACT WITH ASPIRIN

ENOLIC ACIDS
    Piroxicam   (Feldene)
CARBOXYLIC ACIDS
    Acetic acids
        Indomethacin (Indocin)
        Sulindac (Clinoril)
        Tolmetin (Tolectin)
        Zomepirac (Zomax)
PROPRIONIC ACIDS
    Ibuprofen (Motrin, Rufen)
    Naproxen (Naprosyn)
    Naproxen sodium (Anaprox)
    Fenoprofen (Nalfon)
FENAMATES
    Meclofenamate (Meclomen)
    Mefenamic acid (Ponstel)
SALICYLATES
    Acetylsalicylic acid
      (Aspirin, Easpirin, Zorprin)

Modified from: *Allergy Principles and Practice*,
Middleton E Jr, Reed CE, Ellis EF, Adkinson NF, Yunginger JW
(eds), 3rd Edition, C.V. Mosby Company, St. Louis, 1988,
pp.1544.

CHAPTER II

CARDIOLOGY

FREQUENTLY USED ABBREVIATIONS

AI	AORTIC INSUFFICIENCY
AR	AORTIC REGURGITATION
AS	AORTIC STENOSIS
ASD	ATRIAL SEPTAL DEFECT
CHD	CONGENITAL HEART DISEASE OR DEFECT
CHF	CONGESTIVE HEART FAILURE
COA	COARCTATION OF THE AORTA
ECD	ENDOCARDIAL CUSHION DEFECT
ECHO	ECHOCARDIOGRAPHY OR ECHOCARDIOGRAPHIC
HLHS	HYPOPLASTIC LEFT HEART SYNDROME
HOCM	HYPERTROPHIC OBSTRUCTIVE CARDIOMYOPATHY
IHSS	IDIOPATHIC HYPERTROPHIC SUBAORTIC STENOSIS
IVC	INFERIOR VENA CAVA
LA	LEFT ATRIUM OR LEFT ATRIAL
LAD	LEFT AXIS DEVIATION
LAH	LEFT ATRIAL HYPERTROPHY
LBBB	LEFT BUNDLE BRANCH BLOCK
LICS	LEFT INTERCOSTAL SPACE
LLSB	LOWER LEFT STERNAL BORDER
LPA	LEFT PULMONARY ARTERY
LPLs	LEFT PRECORDIAL LEADS
LRSB	LOWER RIGHT STERNAL BORDER
LSB	LEFT STERNAL BORDER
LV	LEFT VENTRICLE OR LEFT VENTRICULAR
LVH	LEFT VENTRICULAR HYPERTROPHY
MI	MITRAL INSUFFICIENCY
MLSB	MID-LEFT STERNAL BORDER
MPA	MAIN PULMONARY ARTERY
MR	MITRAL REGURGITATION
MRSB	MID-RIGHT STERNAL BORDER
MS	MITRAL STENOSIS
MVPS	MITRAL VALVE PROLAPSE SYNDROME
PA	PULMONARY ARTERY OR POSTEROANTERIOR
PAC	PREMATURE ATRIAL CONTRACTION
PAPVR	PARTIAL ANOMALOUS PULMONARY VENOUS RETURN
PAT	PAROXYSMAL ATRIAL TACHYCARDIA
PBF	PULMONARY BLOOD FLOW

PDA	PATENT DUCTUS ARTERIOSUS
PR	PULMONARY REGURGITATION
PS	PULMONARY STENOSIS
PV	PULMONARY VEIN OR PULMONARY VENOUS
PVC	PREMATURE VENTRICULAR CONTRACTION
PVM	PULMONARY VASCULAR MARKINGS
PVOD	PULMONARY VASCULAR OBSTRUCTIVE DISEASE
PVR	PULMONARY VASCULAR RESISTANCE
RA	RIGHT ATRIUM OR RIGHT ATRIAL
RAD	RIGHT AXIS DEVIATION
RAH	RIGHT ATRIAL HYPERTROPHY
RBBB	RIGHT BUNDLE BRANCH BLOCK
RICS	RIGHT INTERCOSTAL SPACE
RPA	RIGHT PULMONARY ARTERY
RPLs	RIGHT PRECORDIAL LEADS
RV	RIGHT VENTRICLE OR RIGHT VENTRICLE
RVH	RIGHT VENTRICULAR HYPERTROPHY
S1	FIRST HEART SOUND
S2	SECOND HEART SOUND
S3	THIRD HEART SOUND
S4	FOURTH HEART SOUND
SEM	SYSTOLIC EJECTION MURMUR
SVC	SUPERIOR VENA CAVA
SVR	SYSTEMIC VASCULAR RESISTANCE
TA	TRICUSPID ATRESIA
TAPVR	TOTAL ANOMALOUS PULMONARY VENOUS RETURN
TGA	TRANSPOSITION OF THE GREAT ARTERIES
TOF	TETRALOGY OF FALLOT
TR	TRICUSPID REGURGITATION
TS	TRICUSPID STENOSIS
ULSB	UPPER LEFT STERNAL BORDER
URSB	UPPER RIGHT STERNAL BORDER
VSD	VENTRICULAR SEPTAL DEFECT
WPW	WOLFF-PARKINSON-WHITE

Modified from: *Pediatric Cardiology for Practitioners*, Year Book Medical Publishers, Inc., Chicago, 1988, pp.XIII-XIV.

CRITERIA FOR DIAGNOSING NONPATHOLOGIC HEART MURMURS

SYSTOLIC MURMUR
EJECTION QUALITY
SOFT OR VIBRATORY
INTENSITY LESS THAN GRADE 3/6
NORMAL PHYSIOLOGICALLY SPLIT SECOND
  HEART SOUND
NO EXTRA SOUNDS OR CLICKS ARE PRESENT
NORMAL CARDIAC IMPULSE
    No thrills
    Normal peripheral pulses
NO PHYSICAL STIGMATA COMMONLY ASSOCIATED
  WITH CARDIAC DISEASE (e.g. DOWN)

Modified from: *Difficult Diagnosis in Pediatrics*,
Stockman JA (ed), W.B. Saunders Company, Philadelphia,
1990, p.93.

INNOCENT MURMURS OF CHILDHOOD

PULMONARY FLOW
    Left upper sternal border
    Soft
    Decreases in intensity with sitting
VIBRATORY (STILL'S)
    Left lower sternal border
    Apex
    Vibratory or musical
PERIPHERAL PULMONIC STENOSIS
    Wide radiation
    Often loudest in the back
      or axillae
VENOUS HUM
    Base, particularly on the right
    Continuous
    Loudest at S_2
    Varies with position and
      neck compression

Modified from: *Difficult Diagnosis in Pediatrics*,
Stockman JA (ed), W.B. Saunders Company, Philadelphia,
1990, p.94.

SUMMARY OF THE SECOND HEART SOUND

WIDELY SPLIT AND FIXED S_2
   Volume overload
       ASD
       Partially anomolous pulmonary
          venous return
   Pressure overload
       Pulmonary valvular stenosis
       Pulmonary infundibular stenosis
   Electrical delay
       Right bundle branch block
   Early aortic closure
       Mitral regurgitation
   Occasional normal child
NARROWLY SPLIT S_2
   Pulmonary hypertension
   Aortic stenosis
   Occasional normal child
SINGLE S_2
   A_2 delayed
       Severe AS
   P_2 occurs early
       Pulmonary hypertension
   P_2 not audible
       Transposition of great vessels
       Tetralogy of fallot
       Atretic or severely stenotic
          pulmonary valve
   One semilunar valve
       Pulmonary atresia
       Aortic atresia
       Persistent truncus arteriosus
   Occasional normal child
   Paradoxically split S_2
       Severe AS
       Left bundle branch block
       WPW syndrome (type B)
   Abnormal intensity of P_2
       Increased P_2
          Pulmonary hypertension
       Decreased P_2
          Severe PS
          TOF
          Tricuspid stenosis

Modified from: Park MK. *Pediatric Cardiology for Practitioners*. Year Book Medical Publishers, Chicago, 1988, p.17.

CYANOTIC CONGENITAL HEART DISEASE

"THE FIVE T's AND ONE P"

Transposition of the great arteries
Truncus arteriosus
Tetralogy of Fallot
Total anomalous pulmonary venous
    return
Tricuspid atresia
Pulmonary atresia

CYANOTIC DEFECTS BY PULMONARY BLOOD FLOW (PBF)

INCREASED PBF AND LEFT VENTRICULAR
  HYPERTROPHY (LVH) OR COMBINED
  VENTRICULAR HYPERTROPHY (CVH)
    Persistent truncus arteriosus
    Single ventricle
    TGA plus VSD
INCREASED PBF AND RIGHT VENTRICULAR
  HYPERTROPHY (RVH)
    TGA
    TAPVR
    Hypoplastic left heart syndrome
      (HLHS)
DECREASED PBF AND CVH
    TGA plus PS
    Persistent truncus arteriosus with
      hypoplastic PA
    Single ventricle with PS
DECREASED PBF AND LVH
    Tricuspid atresia
    Pulmonary atresia with
      hypoplastic RV
DECREASED PBF AND RVH
    Tetralogy of Fallot
    Eisenmenger's physiology (secondary
      to ASD, VSD, PDA)
    Ebstein anomaly

Modified from: *Pediatric Cardiology for
Practitioners*, Park MK (ed), 2nd Ed, Year Book
Medical Publishers, Inc., Chicago, 1988, p.62.

REPORTED SITES OF CONNECTION OF TAPVR

LEFT INNOMINATE VEIN
CORONARY SINUS
RIGHT ATRIUM
RIGHT SUPERIOR VENA CAVA
PORTAL SYSTEM
MULTIPLE SITES
UNKNOWN OR OTHER

Modified from: *Moss' Heart Disease in Infants, Children, and Adolescents*, Adams FH, Emmanouilidies GC, Reimenschneider TA (eds), 4th Edition, The Williams & Wilkins Co, Baltimore, 1989, p.587.

ABNORMAL CARDIAC SILHOUETTE

BOOT-SHAPED
     Tetralogy of Fallot
     Tricuspid atresia
EGG ON STRING
     Transposition of the great arteries
SNOWMAN SIGN
     Total anomalous pulmonary venous return

Modified from: Park MK: *Pediatric Cardiology for Practitioners* 2nd Ed, Year Book Medical Publishers, Inc., Chicago, 1988: p.55.

CONDITIONS ASSOCIATED WITH HYPOCHOLESTEROLEMIA

MALNUTRITION
STRICT VEGETARIAN DIET (LOW IN FAT)
INTESTINAL MALABSORPTION
    Celiac disease
    Cystic fibrosis
    Acrodermatitis enteropathica
    Intestinal lymphangiectasia
    Intractable diarrhea
    Other causes of steatorrhea
LIVER DISEASE
    Fulminant hepatic necrosis
    Reye syndrome and other
      hyperammonemic states
    Hepatic parenchymal disease
IMMUNOGLOBULIN DISORDERS
MYELOPROLIFERATIVE DISORDERS
RETICULOENDOTHELIAL SYSTEM PROLIFERATION
    Gaucher disease
    Niemann-Pick disease
    Kala-azar
    Chronic anemia associated
      with splenomegaly
ENDOCRINE DISORDERS
    Diabetes (low HDL)
    Hypothyroidism
    Hyperthyroidism
SEVERE INFECTIONS
    Sepsis
MITRAL VALVE PROLAPSE SYNDROME

Modified from: Granot E, Deckelbaum RJ: *J Pediatr* 115:171-184, 1989.

CONDITIONS AND THEIR ASSOCIATED ECG CHANGES

HYPERKALEMIA (IN ORDER OF APPEARANCE
  WITH INCREASING K^+)
  Tall "peaked" T waves
  Prolongation of QRS duration
  Prolongation of PR interval
  Disappearance of P wave
  Wide, bizarre diphasic QRS
    complex ("sine wave")
  Eventual asystole
HYPOKALEMIA
  Decrease in T wave amplitude
  Prominent U wave
  S-T segment depression
  Diphasic T wave
HYPOCALCEMIA
  Prolonged Q-T interval
HYPERCALCEMIA
  Short Q-T interval
PERICARDITIS
  Acute
      Elevated S-T segment
      Increased amplitude of T-wave
      Lower overall voltage if
        associated with effusion
  Late
      S-T segment returns to normal
      T-wave inversion
MYOCARDIAL INFARCTION
  Hyperacute phase (a few hours)
      Elevated S-T segment
      Deep and wide Q wave
  Early evolving phase (a few days)
      Deep and wide Q wave
      Elevated S-T segment
      Diphasic T wave
  Late evolving phase (2-3 weeks)
      Deep and wide Q wave
      Sharply inverted T wave
  Revolving phase (years)
      Deep and wide Q wave
      Almost normal T wave

HYPOTHYROIDISM
    Non-specific low voltage changes
    Sinus bradycardia (usually after 3
        years of age)
    Mosque sign
        Dome-shaped symmetric T wave
        Absent S-T segment
HYPERTHYROIDISM
    Sinus tachycardia
    Left ventricular hypertrophy
    Less common
        Prolonged P-R interval
        Non-specific ST-T wave changes
        Right bundle branch block
FRIEDREICH'S ATAXIA
    T vector changes in limb leads
        and/or left precordial leads
    Left ventricular hypertrophy
    Right ventricular hypertrophy
    Abnormal Q waves
MUCOPOLYSACCHARIDOSIS
    Prolonged Q-T interval
    Right ventricular hypertrophy
    Left ventricular hypertrophy
    Left atrial hypertrophy
MARFAN SYNDROME
    Left ventricular hypertrophy
    First degree AV block
    Inversion of T wave in leads II,
        III, aVF and V6
DISSEMINATED LUPUS ERYTHEMATOSUS
    Pericarditis
    Flat or inverted T waves
HYPOTHERMIA
    J wave (Osborne wave)
    Prolonged P-R interval
    Prolonged Q-T interval
    S-T segment elevation or depression
    Bradycardia
    Atrial fibrillation

TRICYCLIC ANTIDEPRESSANTS
- Sinus tachycardia
- Prolonged P-R interval
- Flat T waves
- Less common
    - QRS prolongation
    - QT prolongation
    - ST-T wave changes
- Overdose
    - Any atrial or ventricular dysrhythmias
    - AV block

ORGANOPHOSPHATE INGESTION
- Early sympathetic discharge phase
    - Sinus tachycardia
- Parasympathetic discharge phase
    - Sinus bradycardia
    - AV block
- Late phase
    - Prolongation Q-T interval
    - Torsade de Pointes ventricular tachycardia

DIGITALIS THERAPY
- Effects
    - Shortening Q-T interval
    - Sagging S-T segment
    - Diminished amplitude of the T wave
    - Slowing heart rate
- Toxicity
    - Prolongation of PR interval (from baseline) may progress to second degree AV block
    - Profound sinus bradycardia or sinoatrial block
    - Supraventicular dysrhythmias (more common with children)
    - Ventricular arrhythmias

ATHLETE IN PEAK CONDITION
- Voltage changes consistent with LVH and RVH
- T wave inversion in left chest leads
    (this applies to two of the three editors of this book)

Anxiety or hyperventilation
Altered T waves
Drinking ice cold liquids
T wave inversion
Ingestion of heavy meal
T wave inversion of left
chest leads
CRITERIA FOR WOLFF-PARKINSON-WHITE
SYNDROME
Short P-R interval (less than
normal lower limit)*
Delta wave
Wide QRS duration

*Lower limit of normal P-R interval per age

Less than 3 years	0.08 second
3-16 years	0.10 second
More than 16 years	0.12 second

Modified from: Park MK: *Pediatric Cardiology for Practitioners*, 2nd Edition, Year Book Medical Publishers, Inc, Chicago, 1988, pp.255-257, 277-281.

Pediatrics, Rudolph AM, Hoffman JIE (eds), 18th Edition, Appleton & Lange, Norwalk, 1987, p.1236.

SIMPLE FAINT VERSUS OMINOUS SYNCOPAL EPISODE

SIMPLE FAINT

CONDITIONS	Crowds, hunger, heat, dehydration, pain (or perceived pain), emotion
PRIOR WARNING	Prodrome
INJURY FROM FALL	Rare
DURATION	Less than 1 minute
RECURRENCES	Rare

POSSIBLY OMINOUS FAINT

CONDITIONS	During exercise, loud noises, extreme surprise, anger, or no apparent cause
PRIOR WARNING	None or chest pain, fatigue, palpitations
INJURY FROM FALL	May occur
DURATION	Usually longer than 1 minute
RECURRENCES	Occur repeatedly

Modified from: *The Science and Practice of Pediatric Cardiology*, Garson AJ, Bricker JT, McNamara DG (eds), Lea & Febiger, Philadelphia, 1990, p.1931.

ETIOLOGIC CLASSIFICATION OF SYNCOPE

CIRCULATORY CAUSES
    Extracardiac causes
        Common faint (or vasodepressor syncope)
        Orthostatic hypotension
        Failure of venous return
            Increased intrathoracic pressure
            Decreased venous return
            Hypovolemia
            Other
        Cerebrovascular occlusive disease
    Intracardiac causes
        Severe obstructive lesions
            Aortic stenosis
            Pulmonary stenosis
            Hypertrophic obstructive cardiomyopathy
            Pulmonary hypertension
            Other
        Arrhythmias
METABOLIC CAUSES
    Hypoglycemia
    Hyperventilation syndrome
    Hypoxia
NEUROPSYCHIATRIC CAUSES
    Epilepsy
    Brain tumor
    Migraine
    Hysteria or nonconvulsive seizures

Modified from: *Pediatric Cardiology for Practitioners* 2nd Edition, Year Book Medical Publishers, Inc, Chicago, 1988, p.339.

CARDIOVASCULAR EFFECTS OF HIGH ALTITUDE

DECREASES
> Stroke volume
> Cardiac output
> Systemic vascular resistance
> Coronary blood flow

INCREASES
> Heart rate
> Pulmonary vascular resistance

NORMAL
> Contractility

Modified from: *The Science and Practice of Pediatric Cardiology*, Garson A Jr, Bricker JT, McNamara DG (eds), Lea & Febiger, Philadelphia, 1990, p.443.

CAUSES OF CHEST PAIN IN CHILDREN

CARDIAC
> Structural heart defects
>> Severe obstructive lesions (severe AS, PS, HOCM)
>> Pulmonary vascular obstructive disease
>> Mitral valve prolapse (?)
>> Anomalous origin of the coronary artery
> Inflammatory
>> Pericarditis (viral, bacterial, rheumatic)
>> Kawasaki syndrome
> Arrhythmias
>> Supraventricular tachycardia
>> Frequent PVCs or ventricular tachycardia (?)

THORACIC CAGE
> Costochondritis
> Muscle strain or direct trauma to the chest wall

RESPIRATORY
    Severe cough or bronchitis
    Pleural effusion
    Lobar pneumonia
    Spontaneous pneumothorax
    Pleurodynia or other viral
        infection
    Hyperventilation
PSYCHOGENIC
    Hyperventilation
    Conversion symptoms
    Somatization disorder
    Depression

Modified from: *Pediatric Cardiology for Practitioners*, 2nd Edition, Year Book Medical Publishers, Inc, Chicago, 1988, p.337.

ETIOLOGY OF PERSISTENT PULMONARY HYPERTENSION OF THE NEWBORN

PULMONARY VASOCONSTRICTION WITH NORMALLY
    DEVELOPED PULMONARY VASCULAR BED
        Alveolar hypoxia
            Meconium aspiration syndrome
            Hyaline membrane disease
            Hypoventilation due to CNS
                anomalies
        Birth asphyxia
        LV dysfunction or circulatory shock
        Infections (group B streptococcal
            infection)
        Hyperviscosity syndrome
            (polycythemia)
        Hypoglycemia and hypocalcemia
INCREASED PULMONARY VASCULAR SMOOTH
    MUSCLE (HYPERTROPHY) CAUSED BY
        Chronic intrauterine asphyxia
        Maternal use of prostaglandin
            synthesis inhibitors
                Aspirin
                Indomethacin

CARDIOLOGY   29

DECREASED CROSS-SECTIONAL AREA OF PULMONARY
  VASCULAR BED WITH
        Congenital diaphragmatic hernia
        Primary pulmonary hypoplasia

Modified from: *Pediatric Cardiology for Practitioners*
2nd Edition, Year Book Medical Publishers, Inc, Chicago,
1988, p.296.

CAUSES OF MYOCARDIAL INFARCTION IN CHILDREN

ANOMALOUS LEFT CORONARY ARTERY	20.0%
KAWASAKI SYNDROME	14.0%
MYOCARDITIS	13.0%
CRITICAL CONGENITAL AORTIC STENOSIS	11.0%
VENTRICULAR TUMOR	6.1%
DILATED CARDIOMYOPATHY	4.0%
PULMONARY ATRESIA, INTACT VENTRICULAR SEPTUM	4.0%
PERINATAL ASPHYXIA	4.0%
AORTIC THROMBOSIS	4.0%
MUSCULAR DYSTROPHY CARDIOMYOPATHY	2.5%
COARCTATION OF AORTA	2.5%
RHEUMATIC CARDITIS	2.5%
LYMPHOMA	2.5%
TOTAL ANOMALOUS PULMONARY VENOUS CONNECTION	2.5%
MITRAL VALVE PROLAPSE	2.5%
CONGENITAL MITRAL REGURGITATION	2.5%
BLUNT CHEST TRAUMA	2.5%

Modified from: *The Science and Practice of Pediatric
Cardiology*, Garson A Jr, Bricker JT, McNamara DG (eds),
Lea & Febiger, Philadelphia, 1990, p.1712.

CAUSES OF PULMONARY HYPERTENSION (PH)

LARGE LEFT-TO-RIGHT SHUNT LESIONS
("HYPERKINETIC" PH)
- VSD
- PDA
- Endocardial cushion defect (ECD)
- Others

ALVEOLAR HYPOXIA
- Pulmonary parenchymal disease
  - Extensive pneumonia
  - Lung hypoplasia (primary or secondary, e.g., diaphragmatic hernia)
  - Bronchopulmonary dysplasia
  - Interstitial lung disease (Hammon-Rich syndrome)
  - Wilson-Mikity syndrome
- Airway obstruction
  - Upper airway
    - Large tonsils
    - Macroglossia
    - Micrognathia
    - Laryngotracheomalacia
  - Lower airway
    - Bronchial asthma
    - Cystic fibrosis
- Inadequate ventilatory drive (CNS disease)
- Disorders of chest wall or respiratory muscle
  - Kyphoscoliosis
  - Weakening or paralysis of skeletal muscle
- High altitude

PULMONARY VENOUS HYPERTENSION
- Mitral stenosis
- Cor triatriatum
- TAPVR with obstruction
- Chronic heart failure
- Left sided obstructive lesions, e.g., AS, COA

PRIMARY PULMONARY VASCULAR DISEASE
- Persistent pulmonary hypertension of the newborn
- Primary pulmonary hypertension - rare
- Eisenmenger's physiology
  - Secondary to long-standing "hyperkinetic" PH
- Thromboembolism
  - Ventriculovenous shunt for hydrocephalus
  - Sickle cell anemia
  - Thrombophlebitis

PORTAL HYPERTENSION
- Portal vein thrombosis
- Liver disease

GRANULOMATOUS DISEASE
- Sarcoidosis

COLLAGEN VASCULAR DISEASE
- Rheumatoid arthritis
- Systemic lupus erythematosus
- Scleroderma
- Mixed connective tissue disease

DRUGS
- Aminorex

UNEXPLAINED
- Arterial abnormality
- Venous abnormality

Modified from: *Pediatric Cardiology for Practitioners* 2nd Edition, Year Book Medical Publishers, Inc, Chicago, 1988, p.296.

Moss' Heart Disease in Infants, Children, and Adolescents, Emmanouilides GC, Riemenschneider TA (eds), 4th Edition, The Williams & Wilkins Co, Baltimore, 1989, p.856.

PRIMARY CAUSES OF CARDIOMYOPATHY IN CHILDREN

> DILATED
>> Idiopathic dilated cardiomyopathy
>> Endocardial fibroelastosis
>
> HYPERTROPHIC
>> Obstructive
>> Nonobstructive
>
> RESTRICTIVE
>> Endomyocardial fibrosis
>> Löffler eosinophilic endomyocardial disease
>> Hemochromatosis
>> Fabry disease
>> Pseudoxanthoma elasticum
>
> ARRHYTHMOGENIC
>> Arrhythmogenic right ventricular dysplasia
>> Oncocytic cardiomyopathy

Modified from: *Principles and Practice of Pediatrics*, Oski FA (ed), Lippincott, Philadelphia, 1990, p.1467.

INDICATIONS FOR ANTIBIOTIC PROPHYLAXIS TO PREVENT ENDOCARDITIS*

> PROPHYLAXIS RECOMMENDED
>> Prosthetic cardiac valves (including biosynthetic valves)
>> Most congenital cardiac malformations
>> Surgically constructed systemic-pulmonary shunts
>> Rheumatic, calcific, or other acquired valvular dysfunction
>> Idiopathic hypertrophic subaortic stenosis (IHSS)
>> Previous history of bacterial endocarditis
>> Mitral valve prolapse with mitral insufficiency
>> Postoperative patients (repair or palliation)

CONTROVERSIAL
    Ventriculoatrial shunts for
      hydrocephalus
    Dialysis fistulae and shunts
    Transvenous pacemakers
PROPHYLAXIS NOT RECOMMENDED
    Isolated secundum atrial septal defect
    Secundum atrial septal defect repaired
      without a patch at least six months
      earlier
    Patent ductus arteriosus ligated and
      divided at least six months earlier

*   This list contains common conditions and is
     not meant to be all inclusive.

Modified from: Committee on Prevention of Rheumatic Fever
and Bacterial Endocarditis of the American Heart
Association: *Prevention of Bacterial Endocarditis*.
Circulation 70:1123A-1128A, 1984.

ETIOLOGIC AGENTS OF MYOCARDITIS

VIRAL
  Coxsackievirus A
  Coxsackievirus B
  Echoviruses
  Rubella virus
  Measles virus
  Adenoviruses
  Polio viruses
  Vaccinia virus
  Mumps virus
  Herpes-simplex virus
  Epstein-Barr virus
  Cytomegalovirus
  Rhinoviruses
  Hepatitis viruses
  Arboviruses
  Influenza viruses
  Varicella virus
RICKETTSIAL
  Rickettsia ricketsii
  Rickettsia tsutsugamushi
BACTERIAL
  Meningococcus
  Klebsiella
  Leptospira
  Diphtheria
  Salmonella
  Clostridia
  Tuberculosis
  Brucella
  Legionella pneumophilia
  Streptococcus
PROTOZOAL
  Trypanosoma cruzi
  Toxoplasmosis
  Amebiasis
OTHER PARASITES
  Toxocara canis
  Shistosomiasis
  Heterophyiasis
  Cysticercosis
  Echinococcus
  Visceral larva migrans

FUNGI AND YEASTS
    Actinomycosis
    Coccidiomycosis
    Histoplasmosis
    Candida
TOXIC
    Scorpion
DRUGS
    Sulfonamides
    Phenylbutazone
    Cyclophosphamide
    Neomercazole
    Acetazolamide
    Amphotericin B
    Indomethacin
    Tetracycline
    Isoniazid
    Methyldopa
    Phenytoin
    Penicillin
HYPERSENSITIVITY/AUTOIMMUNE
    Rheumatoid arthritis
    Rheumatic fever
    Ulcerative colitis
    Systemic lupus erythematosus
OTHER
    Sarcoidosis
    Scleroderma
    Cornstarch
    Idiopathic

Modified from: *Principles and Practice of Pediatrics*,
Oski FA, DeAngelis CD, Feigin RD, Warshaw JB (eds),
Lippincott, Philadelphia, 1990, p.1459.

SECONDARY CAUSES OF CARDIOMYOPATHIES

INFECTIONS
    Viral
        Coxsackie B
        Echo
        Mumps
        Rubella
        Rubeola
    Bacterial
        Diphtheria
        Meningococcal
        Pneumococcal
        Gonococcal
    Fungal
        Candidiasis
        Aspergillosis
    Protozoal
        American Trypanosomiasis
          (Chagas disease)
        Toxoplasmosis
    Rickettsial
        Rocky Mountain spotted fever
    Spirochetal
        Lyme disease
METABOLIC CONDITIONS
    Endocrine
        Thyrotoxicosis
        Hypothyroidism
        Diabetes mellitus
            Infant of diabetic mother
            Diabetic cardiomyopathy
        Hypoglycemia
        Pheochromocytoma/neuroblastoma
            Catecholamine
              cardiomyopathy
    Familial storage disease
        Glycogen storage disease
            Pompe disease (Type II)
            Cori disease (Type III)
            Andersen disease (Type
              IV)
            McArdle disease (Type V)
            Hers disease (Type VI)

Mucopolysaccharidoses
    Hurler syndrome
    Hunter syndrome
    Sanfillipo syndrome
    Morquio syndrome
    Scheie syndrome
    Maroteaux-Lamy syndrome
Sphingolipidoses
    Niemann-Pick disease
    Farber disease
    Fabry disease
    Gaucher disease
    Tay-Sachs disease
    Sandhoff disease
    Gm_1 gangliosidosis
    Refsum disease
Nutritional deficiency
    Protein: Kwashiorkor
    Thiamine: Beriberi
    Vitamin E and selenium (Keshan
        disease)
    Phosphate
Others
    Carnitine deficiency
        Primary
        Secondary: diphtheritic
            cardiomyopathy
    B-ketothiolase deficiency
    Hypertaurinuria
GENERAL SYSTEM DISEASES
    Connective tissue disorders
        Systemic lupus erythematosus
        Juvenile rheumatoid arthritis
        Polyarteritis nodosa
        Kawasaki syndrome
        Pseudoxanthoma elasticum
    Infiltrations and granulomas
        Leukemia
        Sarcoidosis (not in children)
        Amyloidosis (not in children)
    Others
        Hemolytic-uremic syndrome
        Mitochondrial cytopathy
        Reye syndrome
        Peripartum cardiomyopathy
        Osteogenesis imperfecta
        Noonan syndrome

HEREDOFAMILIAL CONDITIONS
    Muscular dystrophies and myopathies
        Juvenile progressive
            (Duchenne)
        Myotonic dystrophy (Steinert)
        Limb-girdle (Erb)
        Juvenile progressive spinal
            muscular atrophy
            (Kugelberg-Welander)
        Chronic progressive external
            ophthalmoplegia (Kearns)
        Nemaline myopathy
        Myotubular myopathy
    Neuromuscular disorders
        Friedreich ataxia
        Multiple lentiginosis
SENSITIVITY AND TOXIC REACTIONS
    Sulfonamides
    Penicillin
    Anthracyclines
    Iron (hemachromatosis)
    Chloramphenicol
TACHYARRHYTHMIAS
    Supraventricular tachycardia
    Atrial flutter
    Ventricular tachycardia

Modified from: *The Science and Practice of Pediatric Cardiology*, Garson A Jr, Bricker JT, McNamara DG (eds), Lea & Febiger, Philadelphia, 1990, p.1618.

CARDIOVASCULAR MALFORMATIONS ASSOCIATED WITH CONGENITAL RUBELLA

PULMONARY ARTERIAL STENOSES (COMMON)
PATENT DUCTUS ARTERIOSUS (COMMON)
PULMONARY VALVULAR STENOSIS
SYSTEMIC ARTERIAL STENOSES
HYPOPLASIA OF THE ABDOMINAL AORTA
VENTRICULAR SEPTAL DEFECT

ATRIAL SEPTAL DEFECT
TETRALOGY OF FALLOT
COARCTATION OF THE AORTA
AORTIC VALVULAR OR SUPRAVALVULAR
   STENOSIS
TRANSPOSITION OF THE GREAT ARTERIES
TRICUSPID ATRESIA
MULTIPLE VALVULAR SCLEROSIS

Modified from: *Moss' Heart Disease in Infants, Children, and Adolescents*, Adams FH, Emmanouilides GC, Riemenschneider TA (eds), 4th Edition, The Williams & Wilkins Company, Baltimore, 1989, p.333.

AUTOSOMAL RECESSIVE SYNDROMES/DISORDERS WITH ASSOCIATED CARDIOVASCULAR FINDINGS

ADRENOGENITALISM
      Hyperkalemia
      Broad QRS
      Arrhythmias
ALKAPTONURIA
      Atherosclerosis
      Valvular disease
CARPENTER
      PDA
CONRAD
      VSD
      PDA
COCKAYNE
      Accelerated atherosclerosis
CUTIS LAXA
      Pulmonary hypertension
      Peripheral pulmonary artery stenosis
ELLIS-VAN CREVELD
      ASD
      Single atrium
      Other
FRIEDREICH ATAXIA
      Myocardiopathy
GLYCOGENOSIS IIa, IIIa, AND IV
      Myocardiopathy
HOMOCYSTINURIA
      Coronary and other vascular thromboses

JERVELL-LANGE-NIELSEN
    Prolonged Q-T
    Sudden death
KARTAGENER
    Situs inversus
LAURENCE-MOON-BIEDL
    VSD
    Other
MUCOLIPIDOSIS III
    Aortic valve disease
MUCOPOLYSACCHARIDOSIS (MPS)
    Coronary artery disease
    Aortic insufficiency
    Mitral insufficiency
OSTEOGENESIS IMPERFECTA
    Aortic valve disease
PROGERIA
    Accelerated atherosclerosis
PSEUDO-XANTHOMA ELASTICUM
    Coronary insufficiency
    Mitral insufficiency
    Hypertension
RILEY-DAY
    Episodic hypertension
    Postural hypotension
REFSUM
    Atrioventricular conduction defects
SECKEL
    VSD
    PDA
SICKLE CELL DISEASE
    Myocardiopathy
    Mitral insufficiency
SMITH-LEMLI-OPITZ
    VSD
    PDA
    Other
THROMBOCYTOPENIA AND ABSENT RADIUS (TAR)
    ASD
    TOF
    Dextrocardia

THALASSEMIA MAJOR
    Myocardiopathy
WEILL-MARCHESANI
    PDA
WERNER
    Vascular sclerosis
ZELLWEGER
    PDA
    VSD

Modified from: *Moss' Heart Disease in Infants, Children, and Adolescents*, Adams FH, Emmanouilides GC, Riemenschneider TA (eds), 4th Edition, The Williams & Wilkins Co, Baltimore, 1989, p.17.

The Science and Practice of Pediatric Cardiology, Garson A Jr, Bricker JT, McNamara DG (eds), Lea & Febiger, Philadelphia, 1990, p.2430.

AUTOSOMAL DOMINANT SYNDROME WITH ASSOCIATED CARDIOVASCULAR FINDINGS

ALAGILLE
    Peripheral pulmonary stenosis
    ASD
    VSD
    PDA
    Coarctation of aorta
APERT
    VSD
    TOF
    Crouzon disease
    PDA
    Coarctation of the aorta
EHLERS-DANLOS
    Rupture of large blood vessels
        (e.g., carotids, dissecting aneurysms
        of the aorta)
FAMILIAL PERIODIC PARALYSIS
    Hypokalemia
    Supraventricular tachycardia
FORNEY
    Mitral insufficiency
HOLT-ORAM
    ASD
    VSD

IDIOPATHIC HYPERTROPHIC SUBAORTIC
  STENOSIS (IHSS)
        Subaortic muscular hypertrophy
LEOPARD
        Pulmonary stenosis
        Prolonged P-R interval
        Abnormal P waves
LYMPHEDEMA (MILROY AND MEIGE)
        Lymphedema
MARFAN
        Great artery aneurysms
        Aortic insufficiency
        Mitral insufficiency
MYOTONIC-DYSTROPHY (STEINERT)
        Myocardiopathy
NEUROFIBROMATOSIS
        Pulmonary stenosis
        Pheochromocytoma with hypertension
NOONAN
        PS
        ASD
        IHSS
OSLER-WEBER-RENDU
        Multiple telangiectasias
        Pulmonary arteriovenous fistulas
OSTEOGENESIS IMPERFECTA
        Aortic insufficiency
ROMANO-WARD
        Prolonged Q-T
        Sudden death
TREACHER COLLINS
        VSD
        PDA
        ASD
TUBEROUS SCLEROSIS
        Myocardial rhabdomyoma
VON HIPPEL-LINDAU
        Hemangiomas
        Pheochromocytoma with hypertension

Modified from: *Moss' Heart Disease in Infants,
Children, and Adolescents*, Adams FH, Emmanouilides
GC, Riemenschneider TA (eds), 4th Edition, The Williams
& Wilkins Co, Baltimore, 1989, p.18.

The Science and Practice of Pediatric Cardiology,
Garson A Jr, Bricker JT, McNamara DG (eds), Lea &
Febiger, Philadelphia, 1990, pp.2429-2430.

OTHER CONGENITAL SYNDROMES WITH CONGENITAL HEART DISEASE

DOWN SYNDROME (TRISOMY 21)
- ASD
- VSD
- Cushion defect
- PDA
- Aberrant subclavian artery
- Absent radial artery

TURNER SYNDROME (MONOSOMY XO)
- Coarctation of the aorta
- Bicuspid aortic valve
- Valvular aortic stenosis

EDWARD (TRISOMY 18)
- VSD
- ASD
- PDA
- Bicuspid aortic and pulmonary valves
- Pulmonary stenosis
- Coarctation of the aorta

PATAU (TRISOMY 13)
- VSD
- ASD
- PDA
- Dextroposition
- TAPVR
- Overriding aorta
- Pulmonary stenosis
- Hypoplastic aorta
- Mitral and aortic valve atresia
- Bicuspid aortic valve

TRISOMY 9 MOSAIC
- PDA
- Bicuspid valve
- Tricuspid valve

RUBENSTEIN-TAYBI
- VSD
- PDA
- ASD

DiGEORGE
- Right aortic arch
- Interrupted aorta
- Truncus arteriosus
- VSD
- PDA
- Tetralogy of Fallot

VATER
    VSD
BECKWITH-WIEDEMANN
    Cardiomyopathy
    Hamartomata
INFANT OF A DIABETIC MOTHER
    Hypoplastic right heart
    Hypoplastic left heart
    VSD
    ASD
    Coarctation of the aorta
    Transposition of the great vessels
    Cardiomyopathy
CHARGE
    Tetralogy of Fallot
    PDA
    Double outlet right ventricle
    AV canal
    VSD
    ASD
    Right aortic arch

Modified from: *The Science and Practice of Pediatric Cardiology*, Garson A Jr, Bricker JT, McNamara DG (eds), Lea & Febiger, Philadelphia, 1990, pp.2429-2430.

The Science and Practice of Pediatric Cardiology, Garson A Jr, Bricker JT, McNamara DG (eds), Lea & Febiger, Philadelphia, 1990, p.2498.

FEATURES OF MARFAN SYNDROME

SKELETAL
    Tall stature
    Long arms and legs
      (dolichostenomelia)
    Long fingers (arachnodactyly)
    Narrow, high-arched palate
    Joint hyperextensibility
    Pectus deformity
    Scoliosis
    Congenital contractures

OCULAR
    Flat cornea
    Myopia
    Subluxation of lens (ectopia
        lentis)
    Retinal detachment
PULMONARY
    Pneumothorax
CARDIOVASCULAR
    Ascending aorta dilatation
    Mitral valve prolapse
    Mitral regurgitation
    Aortic regurgitation
    Aortic dissection
    Dysrhythmia
SKIN
    Striae distensae
    Inguinal hernia
CENTRAL NERVOUS SYSTEM
    Dural extasia
    Sacral meningocele
    Dilated cisterna magna

REQUIREMENTS FOR DIAGNOSIS:

If family history is positive, features
in at least two systems listed above
should be present.
If family history is negative for
affected first-degree relative, skeletal
features plus features in at least two
other systems should be present.
Negative nitroprusside test for
homocystinuria.

Modified from: *The Science and Practice of Pediatric Cardiology*, Garson A Jr, Bricker JT, McNamara DG (eds), Lea & Febiger, Philadelphia, 1990, p.2399.

INCIDENCE OF CARDIAC ANOMALIES IN THE OFFSPRING OF A PARENT WITH A CONGENITAL HEART DEFECT

DEFECT	IF MOTHER AFFECTED (%)	IF FATHER AFFECTED (%)
Aortic stenosis	13.0–18.0	3.0
Atrial septal defect	4.0–4.5	1.5
Atrioventricular canal	14.0	1.0
Coarctation of aorta	4.0	2.0
Patent ductus arteriosus	3.5–4.0	2.5
Pulmonary stenosis	4.0–6.5	2.0
Tetralogy of Fallot	6.0–10.0	1.5
Ventricular septal defect	6.0	2.0

Modified from: *Moss' Heart Disease in Infants, Children, and Adolescents*, Adams FH, Emmanouilides GC, Riemenschneider TA (eds), 4th Edition, The Williams & Wilkins Co, Baltimore, 1989, p.20.

RECURRENCE RISKS GIVEN ONE SIBLING WHO HAS A CARDIOVASCULAR ANOMALY

ANOMALY	SUGGESTED RISK %
VSD	3.0
PDA	3.0
ASD	2.5
TOF	2.5
PS	2.0
COA	2.0
AS	2.0
TGA	1.5
AV canal	2.0
Endocardial fibroelastosis	4.0
Ebstein anomaly	1.0
Truncus arteriosus	1.0
PA	1.0
Hypoplastic left heart	2.0

Modified from: *Moss' Heart Disease in Infants, Children, and Adolescents*, Adams FH, Emmanouilides GC, Riemenschneider TA (eds), 4th Edition, The Williams & Wilkins Co, Baltimore, 1989, p.19.

SOME POTENTIAL CARDIOVASCULAR TERATOGENS
(FREQUENCY OF CV DISEASE IN %)

ALCOHOL (25-30)
    VSD
    PDA
    ASD
AMPHETAMINES (?5)
    VSD
    PDA
    ASD
    TGA
ANTICONVULSANTS
    Hydantoin (2-3)
        PS
        AS
        COA
        PDA
    Trimethadione (15-30)
        TGA
        TOF
        HLHS
CHEMOTHERAPY (?5)
    PS
    AS
    VSD
    ASD
LITHIUM (10)
    Ebstein
    TA
    ASD
SEX HORMONES (2-4)
    VSD
    TGA
    TOF
THALIDOMIDE (5-10)
    TOF
    VSD
    ASD
    Truncus arteriosus
RETINOIC ACID (10)
    VSD

Modified from: *Moss' Heart Disease in Infants, Children, and Adolescents*, Adams FH, Emmanouilides GC, Riemenschneider TA (eds), 4th Edition, The Williams & Wilkins Co, Baltimore, 1989, p.20.

DEFECTS INSURABLE AT STANDARD RATES

        ATRIAL SEPTAL DEFECT
            Postoperative
        MITRAL VALVE PROLAPSE WITHOUT
          REGURGITATION
        PATENT DUCTUS ARTERIOSUS
            Postoperative
        PULMONARY STENOSIS, MILD
        PULMONARY STENOSIS
            Postoperative
        HISTORY OF RHEUMATIC FEVER, NO CARDITIS
        VENTRICULAR SEPTAL DEFECT
            Postoperative

Modified from: *Moss' Heart Disease in Infants,
Children, and Adolescents*, Adams FH, Emmanouilides
GC, Riemenschneider TA (eds), 4th Edition, The Williams
& Wilkins Co, Baltimore, 1989, pp.671-672.

DEFECTS INSURABLE AT INCREASED RATES

        AORTIC INSUFFICIENCY
            Mild
            Moderate
        DYSRHYTHMIA
            Sinus node dysfunction
            Supraventricular tachycardia
            Ventricular dysrhythmias
            Congenital complete heart block
        AORTIC STENOSIS
            Mild
            Moderate
            Postoperative
            Subvalvular, mild
            Subvalvular, postoperative
        ATRIAL SEPTAL DEFECT, SMALL
        COARCTATION OF THE AORTA
            Mild
            Postoperative with normal BP
        DEXTROTRANSPOSITION OF THE GREAT
          ARTERIES
            Postoperative
        ENDOCARDIAL CUSHION DEFECT
            Postoperative with no symptoms
            Postoperative with mild mitral
              insufficiency

LEVOTRANSPOSITION OF THE GREAT ARTERIES
    Postoperative
MITRAL INSUFFICIENCY
    Mild
    Moderate
MITRAL VALVE PROLAPSE WITH MILD MITRAL
    INSUFFICIENCY
HISTORY OF RHEUMATIC FEVER WITH MITRAL
    OR AORTIC INSUFFICIENCY
TOTAL ANOMALOUS PULMONARY VENOUS
    CONNECTION
TETRALOGY OF FALLOT
    Postoperative
VENTRICULAR SEPTAL DEFECT
    Small
    Large
    Postoperative with residual shunt

Modified from: *Moss' Heart Disease in Infants, Children, and Adolescents*, Adams FH, Emmanouilides GC, Riemenschneider TA (eds), 4th Edition, The Williams & Wilkins Co, Baltimore, 1989, pp.671-672.

DEFECTS NOT INSURABLE

AORTIC INSUFFICIENCY, SEVERE
ATRIAL SEPTAL DEFECT
    Large
    Postoperative with sinus node
      dysfunction
COARCTATION OF THE AORTA
    Moderate
    Severe
    Postoperative with residual
      hypertension
DEXTROTRANSPOSITION OF THE GREAT
  ARTERIES, PREOPERATIVE EBSTEIN ANOMALY
    Mild
    Moderate
ENDOCARDIAL CUSHION DEFECT
    Unoperated
IDIOPATHIC HYPERTROPHIC SUBAORTIC
  STENOSIS
LEVOTRANSPOSITION OF THE GREAT ARTERIES
    Unoperated
    Postoperative with dysrhythmias
MITRAL VALVE PROLAPSE WITH DYSRHYTHMIAS
PATENT DUCTUS ARTERIOSUS
    Preoperative
PULMONARY STENOSIS, MODERATE
TRICUSPID ATRESIA
TETRALOGY OF FALLOT
    Preoperative
TRUNCUS ARTERIOSUS
VENTRICULAR SEPTAL DEFECT
    Postoperative with residual
      pulmonary vascular occlusive
      disease

Modified from: *Moss' Heart Disease in Infants,
Children, and Adolescents*, Adams FH, Emmanouilides
GC, Riemenschneider TA (eds), 4th Edition, The Williams
& Wilkins Co, Baltimore, 1989, pp.671-672.

CARDIOVASCULAR SURGICAL PROCEDURES

PAB
> Pulmonary artery banding for VSD, severe ASD and large L-R shunts

BLALOCK-HANLON SEPTOSTOMY
> Closed septostomy for TGA

RASHKIND PROCEDURE
> Balloon septostomy for TGA

MUSTARD PROCEDURE
> Epicardial baffle for complete correction TGA

WATERSTON SHUNT
> Ascending aorta anastomosed to R pulmonary artery (for TOF in small infants)

BLALOCK-TAUSSIG
> Subclavian artery anastomosed to pulmonary artery for TOF

GLENN PROCEDURE
> Anastomosis of SVC to R pulmonary artery for tricuspid atresia, TOF?

FANTON "THE FRENCH CONNECTION"
> Anastomose R atrium with pulmonary artery - for tricuspid atresia

STERLING EDWARDS PROCEDURE
> R pulmonary veins to R atrium for TGA

RASTELLI
> Correction of truncus using aortic homograft to connect RV to PA

HANCOCK VALVES
> For correction of pulmonic atresia or truncus

HARDY PROCEDURE
> For Ebstein anomaly, cephalad reposition of tricuspid valve

CONDITIONS ASSOCIATED WITH MITRAL VALVE PROLAPSE

CARDIAC DEFECTS
Congenital heart disease
- Atrial septal defect
- Atrial septal aneurysm
- Ventricular septal defect
- Patent ductus arteriosus
- Tetralogy of Fallot
- Membranous subaortic stenosis
- Aortic valve prolapse
- Bicuspid aortic valve
- Sinus of valsalva aneurysm
- Coarctation
- Tricuspid valve prolapse
- Epstein's anomaly of the tricuspid valve
- Pulmonary stenosis
- Peripheral pulmonary artery stenosis
- Idiopathic dilatation of the pulmonary artery
- Corrected transposition of the great arteries
- Anomalous origin of the LCA from the pulmonary artery
- Coronary artery fistulae
- Coronary ectasia
- Absence of left pericardium

OTHER
- Cardiomyopathy
- Idiopathic hypertrophic cardiomyopathy
- Endomyocardial fibroelastosis
- Left atrial myxoma
- Left ventricular aneurysm
- Atherosclerotic coronary artery disease

CONDUCTION ABNORMALITIES
- Wolff-Parkinson-White syndrome
- Lown-Ganong-Levine syndrome
- Congenital prolonged QT syndrome

CONNECTIVE TISSUE DISEASES
    Marfan syndrome
    Ehlers-Danlos syndrome
    Pseudoxanthoma elasticum
    Osteogenesis imperfecta
    Rheumatoid arthritis
    Raynaud disease
    Mixed connective tissue disease
ENDOCRINE DISORDERS
    Hyperthyroidism
    Chronic thyroiditis
HEMATOLOGIC DISEASES
    Sickle cell disease
    von Willebrand syndrome
    Platelet hypercoagulability
GENETIC
    Turner syndrome
    Noonan syndrome
    Down syndrome
    Duchenne and Berger X-linked muscular
        dystrophy
    Myotonia dystrophy
    Klinefelter syndrome
    Klippel-Feil syndrome
    Fragile X syndrome
THORACIC SPINE AND CHEST WALL ABNORMALITIES
    Pectus excavatum
    Straight-back syndrome
    Women with hypomastia
    Scoliosis
COLLAGEN VASCULAR DISEASE
    Polyarteritis nodosa
    Kawasaki syndrome
    Rheumatic fever
    Systemic lupus erythematosus
METABOLIC DISEASES
    Hunter syndrome
    Hurler syndrome
    Homocystinuria
PULMONARY
    Pulmonary emphysema
    Primary pulmonary hypertension

Modified from: *The Science and Practice of Pediatric Cardiology*, Garson A Jr, Bricker JT, McNamara DG (eds), Lea & Febiger, Philadelphia, 1990, p.1977.

CHAPTER III

DERMATOLOGY

CAUSES OF ACQUIRED DIFFUSE ALOPECIA

ACQUIRED HAIR SHAFT DEFECTS
    Trichorrhexis nodosa
ALOPECIA TOTALIS/UNIVERSALIS
ANAGEN EFFLUVIUM
    Antimitotic agents
    Radiation
    Toxins: thallium, boric acid, lead
TELOGEN EFFLUVIUM
    Physiologic in newborn
    Parturition
    Surgery and anesthesia
    Febrile illness
    Severe dieting
    Drugs
    Endocrine disorders
    Malnutrition

Modified from: *Difficult Diagnosis of Pediatrics*,
Stockman JA III (ed), W.B. Saunders Company,
Philadelphia, 1990, p.272.

CAUSES OF ACQUIRED LOCALIZED ALOPECIA

ALOPECIA AREATA
ANDROGENIC ALOPECIA (MALE PATTERN
  BALDNESS)
DISCOID LUPUS ERYTHEMATOSUS
EPIDERMOLYSIS BULLOSA
FOLLICULAR MUCINOSIS
GRAFT VS HOST DISEASE
LICHEN PLANUS
SCLERODERMA
TINEA CAPITIS
TRAUMATIC ALOPECIA
    Friction
    Injury - burns, radiation,
      chemicals
    Traction
    Trichotillomania

Modified from: *Difficult Diagnosis of Pediatrics*,
Stockman JA III (ed), W.B. Saunders Company,
Philadelphia, 1990, p.272.

CAUSES OF SCARRING ALOPECIA IN CHILDREN

APLASIA CUTIS CONGENITA
DISCOID LUPUS ERYTHEMATOSUS
GRAFT VS HOST DISEASE
INCONTINENTIA PIGMENTI
LICHEN PLANUS
POSTINFECTIOUS: TINEA CAPITIS, HERPES ZOSTER
SCLERODERMA
TRAUMA: BURNS, RADIATION, TRICHOTILLOMANIA

Modified from: *Difficult Diagnosis of Pediatrics*,
Stockman JA III (ed), W.B. Saunders Company, Philadelphia,
1990, p.275.

DRUGS MOST FREQUENTLY CAUSING ALOPECIA

ANTITHYROID DRUGS
ORAL CONTRACEPTIVES
ALKYLATING AGENTS
ANTICOAGULANTS
ANTIMETABOLITES
VITAMIN A
CYTOTOXIC AGENTS
COLCHICINE
ALLOPURINOL
PROPRANOLOL
INDOMETHACIN
LEVODOPA
VALPROATE
HYPOCHOLESTEROLEMIC DRUGS
QUINACRINE
TESTOSTERONE (IN WOMEN)
THALLIUM
HEAVY METALS

Modified from: *Dermatology*, Moschella SL, Hurley HJ
(eds), 2nd Edition, W.B. Saunders Company, Philadelphia,
1985, p.432.

EXOGENOUS CAUSES OF HIRSUITISM

ANABOLIC STEROIDS
ANDROGENIC STEROIDS
CYCLOSPORIN
DANAZOL
DIAMOX
DIAZIDE
DILANTIN
MINOXIDIL
ORAL CONTRACEPTIVES
PENICILLAMINE
PHENOTHIAZINES
PSORALENS

Modified from: Bailey-Pridham DD, Sanfilippo JS:
Pediatric Clinics of North America 36:586, 1989.

DIFFERENTIAL DIAGNOSIS OF ATOPIC DERMATITIS

CONTACT DERMATITIS
SEBORRHEIC DERMATITIS
JUVENILE PLANTAR DERMA
PSORIASIS
TINEAS
ACRODERMATITIS ENTEROPATHICA
SCABIES
HISTIOCYTOSIS-X
WISKOTT-ALDRICH SYNDROME
HYPERIMMUNOGLOBLIN E
PHENYLKETONURIA
ATAXIA-TELANGIECTASIA

AGENTS COMMONLY CAUSING CONTACT DERMATITIS

IRRITANTS
    Acids
    Alkalis
    Bleaches
    Bubble bath
    Detergents
    Feces
    Fiberglass
    Fruit juice
    Saliva

                    Soaps
                    Solvents
                    Sweat
                    Urine
                    Weather (cold or dry)
                    Wool
            ALLERGIC
                    Rhus plants
                    Topical medications
                            Benzocaine
                            Diphenhydramine
                            Ethylenediamine
                            Lanolin
                            Mercuric bichloride
                            Neomycin
                            Para-aminobenzoic acid
                            Thimersal
                            Cosmetics and Perfumes
                                    Balsam of Peru
                                    Paraphenyldiamine
                            Clothing and Shoes
                                    Antioxidants
                                    Formaldehyde
                                    Mercaptobenzothiazole
                                    Potassium dichromate
                                    Thiurams
                            Jewelry-nickel

Modified from: *Ambulatory Pediatric Care*, Dershewitz RA
(ed), J.B. Lippincott, Philadelphia, 1988, p.196.

NUTRITIONAL DEFICIENCIES ASSOCIATED WITH DERMATITIS

            RIBOFLAVIN (B$_2$)
            PYRIDOXINE (B$_6$)
            NIACIN
            BIOTIN
            ZINC

Modified from: *Dermatology*, Moschella SL, Hurley HJ
(eds), 2nd Edition, W.B. Saunders Company, Philadelphia,
1985, p.432.

Dermatology in General Medicine: Textbook and Atlas,
Fitzpatrick TB, Eisen AZ, Wolff K, Freedberg IM, Austen KF
(eds), 3rd Edition, McGraw-Hill Company, New York, 1984,
pp.1601-1613.

CONDITIONS ASSOCIATED WITH CAFÉ-AU-LAIT SPOTS

NEUROFIBROMATOSIS
TUBEROUS SCLEROSIS
ALBRIGHT SYNDROME
BLOOM SYNDROME
ATAXIA-TELANGIECTASIA
RUSSELL SILVER SYNDROME
GAUCHER DISEASE
LESCHKE SYNDROME

Modified from: *Pediatrics*, Rudolph AM (ed), 18th Edition, Appleton & Lange, Norwalk, 1987, p.833.

SYSTEMIC DISEASES ASSOCIATED WITH PHOTOSENSITIVITY

BIOCHEMICAL
    Porphyrias
    Aminoacidurias
    Pellagra
    Albinism
    Hypopituitary and hypogonadal
        disorders
IMMUNOLOGIC
    Systemic lupus erythematosus
    Pemphigus erythematosus
    Dermatomyositis
    Scleroderma
    Vitiligo
    Eczema, photosensitive type
    Reticular erythematosus mucinosis
GENETIC
    Xeroderma pigmentosum
    Bloom syndrome
    Cockayne syndrome
    Rothmund-Thompson syndrome
    Disseminated superficial actinic
        porokeratosis

INFECTIOUS
        Herpes simplex
        Lymphogranuloma venereum

Modified from: *Dermatology*, Moschella SL, Hurley HJ
(eds), 2nd Edition, W.B. Saunders Company, Philadelphia,
1985, pp.403-409.

Dermatology in General Medicine: Textbook and Atlas,
Fitzpatrick TB, Eisen AZ, Wolff K, Freedberg IM, Austen KF
(eds), 3rd Edition, McGraw-Hill Company, New York, 1984,
pp.1481-1506.

CAUSES OF STEVENS-JOHNSON SYNDROME

INFECTIONS
        Viruses
        Fungi
        Bacteria
        Parasites
INGESTANTS
        Drugs
        Food additives and dyes
CONTACTANTS
PHYSICAL FACTORS
        Cold
        Sun
COLLAGEN VASCULAR DISEASES
MALIGNANCY
PREGNANCY

Modified from: *Dermatology*, Moschella SL, Hurley HJ
(eds), 2nd Edition, W.B. Saunders Company, Philadelphia,
1985, p.468.

DRUGS MOST FREQUENTLY CAUSING ERYTHEMA NODOSUM

    IODIDES
    ORAL CONTRACEPTIVES
    PHENACETIN
    SALICYLATES
    SULFONAMIDES
    SULFONES
    PENICILLIN
    BARBITURATES
    HYDANTOIN

Modified from: *Dermatology*, Moschella SL, Hurley HJ
(eds), 2nd Edition, W.B. Saunders Company,
Philadelphia, 1985, p.432.

CAUSES OF BULLOUS ERUPTIONS IN THE NEONATAL PERIOD

    APLASIA CUTIS
    BULLOUS IMPETIGO
    BURNS
    CUTANEOUS MASTOCYTOSIS
    EPIDERMOLYSIS BULLOSA
    EPIDERMOLYTIC HYPERKERATOSIS
    HERPES SIMPLEX
    INCONTINENTIA PIGMENTI
    INSECT BITES
    SCABIES
    SUCKLING BLISTERS
    STAPHYLOCOCCAL SCALDED SKIN SYNDROME

Modified from: *Difficult Diagnosis of Pediatrics*,
Stockman JA III (ed), W.B. Saunders Company,
Philadelphia, 1990, p.268.

DRUGS MOST FREQUENTLY CAUSING URTICARIA

ACTH
BARBITURATES
CHLORAMPHENICOL
GRISEOFULVIN
INDOMETHACIN
INSULIN
OPIATES
PENICILLINS
PHENOLPHTHALEIN
PHENOTHIAZINE
SALICYLATES
STREPTOMYCIN
SULFONAMIDES
TETRACYCLINES

Modified from: *Dermatology*, Moschella SL, Hurley HJ
(eds), 2nd Edition, W.B. Saunders Company, Philadelphia,
1985, p.433.

CAUSES OF DIFFUSE HYPERPIGMENTATION

SUN EXPOSURE
ADDISON DISEASE
NELSON SYNDROME
CUSHING SYNDROME
ACROMEGALY
PREGNANCY
MELANOSIS CACHECTICORUM
VITAMIN DEFICIENCY (B_{12}, FOLATE,
    NIACIN, A, AND ASCORBIC ACID)
HEMOCHROMATOSIS
BILIARY CIRRHOSIS
WILSON DISEASE
VON GIERKE GLYCOGEN STORAGE DISEASE
PORPHYRIA CUTANEA TARDA
SCLERODERMA
RHEUMATOID ARTHRITIS
STILL DISEASE
NIEMANN-PICK DISEASE
FANCONI SYNDROME
GAUCHER DISEASE
DRUGS

Modified from: *Dermatology*, Moschella SL, Hurley HJ
(eds), 2nd Edition, W.B. Saunders Company, Philadelphia,
1985, pp.1282-1285.

CAUSES OF ALLERGIC OR CONTACT VULVOVAGINITIS

SOAPS AND OTHER CLEANING AGENTS
COLORED TOILET PAPER
BUBBLE BATH
CHEMICAL DOUCHES
FEMININE DEODORANT SPRAYS
SPERMICIDES
CONDOM LUBRICANTS
CONTRACEPTIVE JELLY, FOAMS, AND
    SUPPOSITORIES
SANITARY NAPKINS
RAYON OR NYLON UNDERPANTS
OBESITY
HOT WEATHER
POOR HYGIENE
SAND
PERFUMES
LAUNDRY DETERGENTS
MEDICATIONS
DEPILATORIES AND SHAVING CREAMS

Modified from: Rosenfeld WD, Clark J: *Pediatric Clinics of North America* 36:495, 1989.

CHAPTER IV

ENDOCRINOLOGY

CAUSES OF THYROMEGALY

DIFFUSE
- Hashimoto thyroiditis
- Thyrotoxicosis
  - Grave disease
  - Thyroiditis
  - TSH-secreting adenoma
  - Pituitary resistance
- Goitrogen exposure
- Dyshormonogenesis
- Iodine deficiency (endemic)
- Idiopathic (simple) goiter
- Acute, subacute thyroiditis

NODULAR
- Hashimoto thyroiditis
- Thyroid cyst
- Thyroid adenoma
  - Hyperfunctional (hot)
  - Hypofunctional (cold)
- Thyroid carcinoma
  - Papillary
  - Follicular
  - Mixed papillary/follicular
  - Anaplastic
  - Medullary

Modified from: *Principles and Practice of Pediatrics*, Oski FA, DeAngelis CD, Feigin RD, Warshaw JB (eds), J.B. Lippincott, Philadelphia, 1990, p.1823.

SIGNS AND SYMPTOMS OF HYPERTHYROIDISM

GOITER
ANXIOUSNESS, NERVOUSNESS
TACHYCARDIA
WIDE PULSE PRESSURE
INCREASED APPETITE
WEIGHT LOSS OR GAIN
TREMOR
PROPTOSIS
HEAT INTOLERANCE
INCREASED GROWTH VELOCITY
DIARRHEA

Modified from: *Principles and Practice of Pediatrics*,
Oski FA, DeAngelis CD, Feigin RD, Warshaw JB (eds), J.B.
Lippincott, Philadelphia, 1990, p.1822.

SIGNS AND SYMPTOMS OF CONGENITAL HYPOTHYROIDISM

LARGE FONTANELLES
UMBILICAL HERNIA
MACROGLOSSIA
MOTTLED, DRY SKIN
HYPOTONIA
ABDOMINAL DISTENTION
EDEMA
HOARSE CRY
RESPIRATORY SIGNS (APNEA, NOISY RESPIRATIONS,
   NASAL OBSTRUCTION)
ANEMIA
PROLONGED JAUNDICE
CONSTIPATION
LETHARGY
DIFFICULTY FEEDING
COOL SKIN
SLEEPS THROUGH NIGHT (IN NEWBORN PERIOD)
HYPOTHERMIA
GOITER (RARE)
SLOW RELAXATION OF DEEP TENDON REFLEXES

Modified from: *Principles and Practice of Pediatrics*,
Oski FA, DeAngelis CD, Feigin RD, Warshaw JB (eds), J.B.
Lippincott, Philadelphia, 1990, p.1819.

The Thyroid and its Diseases, DeGroot LJ, Larsen PR,
Refetoff S, Stanbury JB (eds), 5th Edition, John Wiley &
Sons, New York City, 1984, p.620.

FACTORS THAT INFLUENCE THYROID BINDING GLOBULIN LEVELS

INCREASED TBG
Congenital (X-Linked)
Hepatitis
Porphyria
Heroin, methadone
Estrogens, pregnancy (oral contraceptives)
5-Fluorouracil
Perphenazine (Trilafon)
DECREASED TBG
Congenital (X-Linked)
Hepatic cirrhosis
Nephrosis
Androgens
Antiestrogens
Glucocorticoids
Acromegaly
Protein-losing enteropathy
Protein-calorie malnutrition
Hyperthyroidism

Modified from: *Principles and Practice of Pediatrics*, Oski FA, DeAngelis CD, Feigin RD, Warshaw JB (eds), J.B. Lippincott, Philadelphia, 1990, p.1817.

SIGNS AND SYMPTOMS OF PHEOCHROMOCYTOMA

HYPERTENSION
SWEATING
PALPITATIONS
TACHYCARDIA
EMOTIONAL LABILITY
HEADACHE
NAUSEA
VOMITING
CONSTIPATION
POLYURIA
POLYDIPSIA

Modified from: *Principles and Practice of Pediatrics*, Oski FA, DeAngelis CD, Feigin RD, Warshaw JB (eds), J.B. Lippincott, Philadelphia, 1990, p.1832.

CLINICAL FEATURES OF HYPERCORTISOLISM
(CUSHING SYNDROME)

OBESITY WITH VIOLACEOUS STRIAE
    Generalized in infants
    Truncal in older children with moon
      facies,
      buffalo hump
DECREASED GROWTH VELOCITY
    Short stature
    Delayed bone age
PLETHORA, INCREASED HEMATOCRIT
HIRSUTISM
MENSTRUAL DISORDERS
HYPERTENSION
MUSCULAR WEAKNESS
MUSCLE WASTING (USUALLY IN INFANTS)
BACK PAIN
ACNE
PSYCHOLOGIC SYMPTOMS
EASY BRUISABILITY
CONGESTIVE HEART FAILURE
EDEMA
HYPERCALCIURIA
RENAL STONES
HEADACHE
POLYURIA-POLYDIPSIA
HYPERPIGMENTATION
OSTEOPOROSIS
POOR WOUND HEALING
GLUCOSE INTOLERANCE
INCREASED FREQUENCY OF INFECTIONS

Modified from: *Principles and Practice of Pediatrics*,
Oski FA, DeAngelis CD, Feigin RD, Warshaw JB (eds), J.B.
Lippincott, Philadelphia, 1990, p.1830.

Basic and Clinical Endocrinology, Greenspan FS, Forsham
PH (eds), 2nd Edition, Appleton-Century-Crofts, East
Norwalk, 1986, p.299.

ETIOLOGY OF ADRENOCORTICAL INSUFFICIENCY

IDIOPATHIC/AUTOIMMUNE
TUBERCULOSIS
VASCULAR
- Hemorrhage
    - Waterhouse-Friderichsen syndrome
    - Anticoagulants
    - Coagulopathy
    - Trauma
    - Surgery
    - Pregnancy
    - Neonate
- Infarction
    - Thrombosis
    - Embolism
    - Arteritis
- FUNGAL INFECTION
    - Histoplasmosis
    - Coccidioidomycosis
    - Blastomycosis
    - Candidiasis
    - Torulosis (Cryptococcosis)

ACQUIRED IMMUNE DEFICIENCY SYNDROME (AIDS)
METASTASES
LYMPHOMA
AMYLOIDOSIS
SARCOIDOSIS
HEMOCHROMATOSIS
IRRADIATION
HEREDITARY CONDITIONS
- Congenital adrenal hyperplasia
- Hypoplasia
- Familial glucocorticoid deficiency

CORTICOTROPIN RELEASING FACTOR DEFICIENCY
CORTICOTROPIN DEFICIENCY
IATROGENIC
- Abrupt cessation of exogenous corticosteroids or corticotropin

DRUGS
- Aminoglutethimide
- Mitotane (O,p-DDD)
- Metyrapone
- Ketaconazole

FEMALE ADRENAL SUPPRESSION - MATERNAL
HYPERCORTISOLISM
Endogenous
Therapeutic

Modified from: *Nelson Textbook of Pediatrics*, Nelson
WE, Behrman RE, Vaughan VC (eds), 13th Edition, W.B.
Saunders Company, Philadelphia, 1987, pp.1215-1220.

Endocrinology and Metabolism, Felig P, Baxter, JD,
Broadus AE, Frohman LA (eds), 2nd Edition, McGraw-Hill Book
Company, New York City, 1987, p.581.

CAUSES OF SHORT STATURE OR POOR LINEAR GROWTH

MAJOR ORGAN SYSTEM DISEASE
CNS
Cardiac
Pulmonary
Hematologic
Renal
Gastrointestinal
MALNUTRITION
CHROMOSOMAL DISORDERS
Turner syndrome
Down syndrome
Females with non-45X karyotypes
INBORN ERRORS OF METABOLISM
INTRAUTERINE GROWTH RETARDATION
FAMILIAL OR GENETIC SHORT STATURE
CONSTITUTIONAL DELAY OF GROWTH AND
ADOLESCENCE
ENDOCRINE DISORDERS
Cortisol excess (exogenous or
endogenous)
Hypothyroidism
Pseudohypoparathyroidism
Poorly controlled diabetes
Growth hormone deficiency
Idiopathic
Organic
Familial
Psychosocial
SHIFTING LINEAR PERCENTILES

SKELETAL DISORDERS
    Rickets
    Deprivation/psychosocial dwarfism
    Lead toxicity
    Medications

Modified from: *Principles and Practice of
Pediatrics*, Oski FA, DeAngelis CD, Feigin RD, Warshaw
JB (eds), J.B. Lippincott, Philadelphia, 1990, p.1830.

Mahoney PC: *Pediatric Clinics of North America*
34:825-849, 1987.

CAUSES OF DELAYED PUBERTY

HYPERGONADOTROPIC CONDITIONS
    Chromosomal abnormalities
        Turner syndrome
        Klinefelter syndrome
    Androgen insensitivity (testicular
        feminization)
    Gonadal failure
        Autoimmune
        Chemotherapy
        Radiation
        Traumatic
        Infectious
        Postsurgical
        Torsion
        "Vanishing testes"
        Pure gonadal dysgenesis
        Myotonic dystrophy
        Galactosemia (females)
    Enzyme blocks
        17 alpha-hydroxylase
            deficiency in the genetic
            male or female
        17-ketosteroid reductase
            deficiency in the genetic
            male
HYPOGONADOTROPIC CONDITIONS
    Constitutional delay of growth and
        adolescence

Hypopituitarism
    Isolated LH/FSH deficiencies
        Associated with hyposmia/
           anosmia (Kallman syndrome)
    Multiple hormone deficiencies
    Panhypopituitarism
Miscellaneous syndrome complexes
    Prader-Willi
    Laurence-Moon-Biedl
Systemic conditions
    Chronic disease
    Malnutrition
    Intensive exercise training
    Psychogenic disorders
    Stress
Other endocrine causes
    Hypothyroidism
    Glucocorticoid excess
    Hyperprolactinemia
Tumors of the hypothalamus or pituitary
    Craniopharyngioma
EUGONADOTROPIC CONDITIONS: DELAYED MENARCHE
    Gonadal dysgenesis variants with
     residually functioning ovarian tissue
    Abnormalities of Müllerian duct
     development
    Polycystic ovarian disease
    Hyperprolactinemia

Modified from: *Principles and Practice of Pediatrics*, Oski FA, DeAngelis CD, Feigin RD, Warshaw JB (eds), J.B. Lippincott, Philadelphia, 1990, pp.1802-1803.

Endocrinology, DeGroot LJ, Besser GM, Cahill GF, et al (eds), 2nd Edition, W.B. Saunders Company, Philadelphia, 1989, pp.1873-1878.

CAUSES OF PRECOCIOUS PUBERTY

PREMATURE ACTIVATION OF GONADOTROPIN
SECRETION (CENTRAL PRECOCIOUS PUBERTY)
- Idiopathic
- CNS tumors (hypothalamic hamartomas, others)
- CNS trauma
- Post infectious
    - Meningitis
    - Encephalitis
- Hydrocephalus
- Neurofibromatosis
- Tuberous sclerosis
- Russell-Silver syndrome
- Severe primary hypothyroidism (untreated)

GONADOTROPIN SECRETION INDEPENDENT
- Girls
    - Exogenous estrogen exposure
    - Estrogen-secreting tumors (adrenals or ovaries)
    - Ovarian cysts
    - McCune-Albright syndrome
- Boys
    - Exogenous androgen exposure
    - Adrenal androgen secretion
        - Congenital adrenal hyperplasia
        - Adrenal tumors
    - Testicular androgen secretion
        - Tumors
        - Familial Leydig cell hyperplasia
    - Gonadotropin-secreting tumors
    - McCune-Albright syndrome

Modified from: *Principles and Practice of Pediatrics*, Oski FA, DeAngelis CD, Feigin RD, Warshaw JB (eds), J.B. Lippincott, Philadelphia, 1990, pp.1799-1801.

Endocrinology, DeGroot LJ, Besser GM, Cahill GF, et al (eds), 2nd Edition, W.B. Saunders Company, Philadelphia, 1989, pp.1886-1889.

CAUSES OF BREAST MASSES

FIBROADENOMA
JUVENILE (GIANT) FIBROADENOMA
OTHER FIBROADENOMA VARIANTS
VIRGINAL HYPERPLASIA
CYSTOSARCOMA PHYLLOIDES
BREAST ABSCESS
BREAST CYST (INCLUDING FIBROCYSTIC
   BREAST DISEASE AND OTHER BREAST
   MASTOPATHIES)
BREAST CARCINOMA
INTRADUCTAL PAPILLOMA
FAT NECROSIS
LIPOMA
LYMPHANGIOMA
HEMANGIOMA
MISCELLANEOUS
       Nipple adenoma
       Papillomatosis
       Ductal adenocarcinoma
       Mammary duct ectasia
       Intraductal granuloma
       Sclerosing adenosis
       Keratoma of the nipple
       Interstitial fibrosis
       Granular cell myoblastoma
       Angiosarcoma of the breast
       Metastatic disease (e.g. leukemia,
         malignant lymphoma, ovarian
         malignancy, others)
       Neurofibromatosis
       Dermatofibromatosis
       Tuberous mastitis
       Papilloma sarcoidosis
       Hematoma
       Others

Modified from: Greydanus DE, Douglas SP, Farrell EG,
Pediatric Clinics of North America 36:618, 1989.

CAUSES OF GYNECOMASTIA

IDIOPATHIC
FAMILIAL
    Associated with anosmia and
      testicular atrophy
    Reifenstein syndrome
    Associated with hypogonadism and
      a small penis
    Others
KLINEFELTER SYNDROME
MALE PSEUDOHERMAPHRODITISM
TESTICULAR FEMINIZATION SYNDROME
TUMORS
    Seminoma
    Leydig cell tumor
    Teratoma
    Feminizing adrenal tumor
    Hepatoma
    Bronchogenic carcinoma
LEUKEMIA
HEMOPHILIA
LEPROSY
THYROID DYSFUNCTION (HYPER- AND
  HYPOTHYROIDISM)
CIRRHOSIS OF THE LIVER
TRAUMATIC PARAPLEGIA
CHRONIC GLOMERULONEPHRITIS
STARVATION (ON REFEEDING)
MISCELLANEOUS DRUGS
    Amphetamines
    Anabolic steroids
    Birth control pills
    Busulfan (and other chemo-
      therapeutic agents)
    Cimetidine
    Clomiphene
    Corticosteroids
    Digitalis
    Estrogens
    Human chorionic gonadotropin
    Insulin
    Isoniazid (and other anti-
      tuberculosis drugs)
    Marijuana

Methadone
Reserpine
Spironolactone
Testosterone
Tricyclic antidepressants
Others

Modified from: Greydanus DE, Douglas SP, Farrell EG,
Pediatric Clinics of North America 36:634, 1989.

CAUSES OF CENTRAL DIABETES INSIPIDUS

IDIOPATHIC
    CNS tumors
        Craniopharyngioma
        Dysgerminoma
        Pinealoma
        Pituitary tumor
        Metastases to hypothalamus
    Trauma
        Head injury
        Postoperative CNS tumor
          resection
    Granulomatous disease
        Sarcoidosis
        Histiocytosis
    Infections
        Meningitis
        Encephalitis
    Vascular disorders
        Aneurysms
        Infarction
        Sickle cell anemia
        Intraventricular hemorrhage
          (neonate)
    Pregnancy
    Sheehan syndrome
    Familial
        Dominant or recessive
        DIDMOAD syndrome (Wolfran syndrome)

Modified from: *Endocrinology*, DeGroot LJ, Besser GM,
Cahill GF, et al (eds), 2nd Edition, W.B. Saunders Company,
Philadelphia, 1989, pp.220-221.

Nelson Textbook of Pediatrics, Nelson WE, Behrman RE,
Vaughan VC (eds), 13th Edition, W.B. Saunders Company,
Philadelphia, 1987, pp.1181-1182.

CAUSES OF HYPERCALCEMIA

HYPERPARATHYROIDISM
    Isolated
    Multiple endocrine neoplasia
        syndrome
NON-PTH MEDIATED
    Ingestions
        Milk-alkali syndrome
        Vitamin D intoxication
        Vitamin A intoxication
        Thiazide diuretics
    Immobilization
    Infection
        Tuberculosis
    Infiltrative
        Sarcoidosis
    Iatrogenic
        Hyperalimentation
    Infantile
        Subcutaneous fat necrosis
        Secondary to maternal
            hypoparathyroidism
        Idiopathic hypercalcemia of
            infancy
        Hyperplasia
        Idiopathic
        Tumors
        Hematogenous malignancy
        Carcinomas of breast, lung,
            multiple myeloma
        Tumors of head, neck, kidney,
            and reproductive organs
        Pheochromocytoma
        Islet cell tumor of the
            pancreas
    Familial hypocalciuria
    Endocrine
        Hyperthyroidism
        Adrenal insufficiency
    Renal failure
        Acute, with rhabdomyolysis
        Chronic

Modified from: Kainer G, Chan JCM: *Current Problems
in Pediatrics*, 19:523-533, 1989.

CHAPTER V

GASTROENTEROLOGY

AGENTS WHICH DECREASE LOWER ESOPHAGEAL SPHINCTER (LES) PRESSURE

ALPHA-ADRENERGIC ANTAGONISTS
ANTICHOLINERGICS
BETA-ADRENERGIC AGONISTS
CAFFEINE
CALCIUM-CHANNEL BLOCKERS
CHOCOLATE
CHOLECYSTOKININ
DEMEROL (OPIATES)
DOPAMINE
ETHANOL
FAT MEAL
GASTRIC ACIDIFICATION
GASTRIC INHIBITORY PEPTIDE
GLUCAGON
PROSTAGLANDINS
SECRETIN
SMOKING
THEOPHYLLINE
VALIUM
VASOACTIVE INTESTINAL PEPTIDE

Modified from: *Textbook of Pediatric Gastroenterology*, Silverberg M, Daum F (eds), 2nd Edition, Year Book Medical Publishers, Inc., Chicago, 1988, p.158.

DRUGS THAT MAY CAUSE HEPATITIS

ACETAMINOPHEN
ALCOHOL
ALLOPURINOL
AMIODARONE
ANABOLIC STEROIDS
AZATHIOPRINE
CARBAMAZEPINE
CIMETIDINE
COCAINE
CYCLOPHOSPHAMIDE
CYCLOSPORIN
DISULFIRAM
ERYTHROMYCIN
GENTAMICIN
HALOTHANE
ISOFLURANE

ISONIAZIDE
KETOCONAZOLE
6-MERCAPTOPURINE
METHOTHREXATE
NIFEDIPINE
NON-STEROIDAL ANTI-
    INFLAMMATORY DRUGS
ORAL CONTRACEPTIVES
PENICILLAMINE
PHENOBARBITAL
PHENOTHIAZINES
PHENYTOIN
PROPYLTHIOURACIL
PYRAZINAMIDE
QUINIDINE
RIFAMPIN

SULFASALAZINE	VALPROIC ACID
SULFONAMIDES	VERAPAMIL
TESTOSTERONE	VINCRISTINE
TETRACYCLINE	

Modified from: AMA Drug Evaluations, 5th Edition, Chicago.

ETIOLOGIES OF FULMINANT HEPATIC FAILURE IN CHILDHOOD

VIRAL INFECTIONS
>   Hepatitis A
>   Hepatitis B
>   Hepatitis non-A, non-B

DRUGS
>   Acetaminophen
>   Halothane
>   Isoniazid
>   Methyldopa
>   Sodium valproate
>   Tetracycline

TOXINS
>   Amanita phalloides
>   Carbon tetrachloride
>   Phosphorous

SYSTEMIC
>   Alpha-1-antitrypsin deficiency
>   Ischemia
>   Leukemia/lymphoma
>   Wilson disease

Modified from: *Manual of Pediatric Gastroenterology*, Fitzgerald JF, Clark JH (eds), Churchill Livingstone, New York City, 1988, p.158.

ETIOLOGIES OF CIRRHOSIS

ALPHA-1 ANTITRYPSIN DEFICIENCY
AUTOIMMUNE
DRUGS AND TOXINS
BILIARY ATRESIA
CHOLEDOCHAL CYST
CONGENITAL HEPATIC FIBROSIS
CYSTIC FIBROSIS
GALACTOSEMIA
GLYCOGEN STORAGE DISEASE
HEMOCHROMATOSIS
HEREDITARY FRUCTOSE INTOLERANCE
INFECTIOUS HEPATITIS
INTRAHEPATIC BILE DUCT PAUCITY
OSLER-WEBER-RENDU DISEASE
SCLEROSING CHOLANGITIS
SEGMENTAL DILATATION OF THE INTRAHEPATIC
   BILIARY TREE
TYROSINEMIA
WILSON DISEASE

Modified from: *Principles and Practice of Pediatrics*, Oski FA, DeAngelis CD, Feigin RD, Warshaw JB (eds), J.B. Lippincott Company, Philadelphia, 1990, p.1783.

RISK FACTORS ASSOCIATED WITH CHOLELITHIASIS

HEREDITARY SPHEROCYTOSIS
SICKLE CELL DISEASE
THALASSEMIA MAJOR
TOTAL PARENTERAL ALIMENTATION
STARVATION
DEHYDRATION
CIRRHOSIS
ILEAL RESECTION
PREGNANCY
ORAL CONTRACEPTIVES
OBESITY
LIVER TRAUMA
PROLONGED IMMOBILIZATION
PREMATURITY
HYALINE MEMBRANE DISEASE
BRONCHOPULMONARY DYSPLASIA
POLYCYTHEMIA
BILIARY TRACT ANOMALIES

Modified from: Holcomb GW Jr, Holcomb GW III: *Pediatrics in Review* 11:268-274, 1990.

FACTORS ASSOCIATED WITH CHOLECYSTITIS

HEMOLYTIC DISEASE
PREGNANCY
OBESITY
INFECTION
FAMILY HISTORY OF BILIARY DISEASE
PREVIOUS ABDOMINAL SURGERY
CYSTIC FIBROSIS
BILIARY TRACT ANOMALIES
CIRRHOSIS
TRAUMA

Modified from: *Principles and Practice of Pediatrics*,
Oski FA, DeAngelis CD, Feigin RD, Warshaw JB (eds), J.B.
Lippincott Company, Philadelphia, 1990, p.1780.

CAUSES OF JAUNDICE BEYOND THE NEONATAL PERIOD

ALAGILLE SYNDROME
ALPHA-1-ANTITRYPSIN DEFICIENCY
BENIGN RECURRENT CHOLESTASIS
BILIARY ATRESIA
BYLER DISEASE
CHEMICAL INJURY
CHOLEDOCHAL CYST
CHOLELITHIASIS
CHRONIC ACTIVE HEPATITIS
CIRRHOSIS
CYSTIC FIBROSIS
DRUG-INDUCED HEPATITIS
DUBIN-JOHNSON SYNDROME
GALACTOSEMIA
GILBERT DISEASE
GLYCOGEN STORAGE DISEASE
HEMOLYTIC ANEMIAS
HEMOPHAGOCYTIC SYNDROMES
HEPATITIS, INFECTIOUS
HEREDITARY FRUCTOSE INTOLERANCE
NIEMANN-PICK DISEASE
PYLORIC STENOSIS
REYE SYNDROME

ROTOR SYNDROME
TOTAL PARENTERAL NUTRITION
TRISOMY 18
TYROSINEMIA
WILSON DISEASE

Modified from: *Principles and Practice of Pediatrics*, Oski FA, DeAngelis CD, Feigin RD, Warshaw JB (eds), J.B. Lippincott Company, Philadelphia, 1990, pp.2044.

CAUSES OF EXOCRINE PANCREATIC INSUFFICIENCY

CYSTIC FIBROSIS
SHWACHMAN SYNDROME
JOHANNSON-BLIZZARD SYNDROME
PROTEIN-CALORIE MALNUTRITION
RELATIVE NEONATAL DEFICIENCY
CHRONIC PANCREATITIS
PEARSON SYNDROME

Modified from: *Manual of Pediatric Gastroenterology*, Fitzgerald JF, Clark JH (eds), Churchill Livingstone, New York City, 1988, p.72.

Practical Paediatric Gastroenterology, Walker-Smith JA, Hamilton JR, Walker WA (eds), Butterworths, London, 1983, p.317.

CAUSES OF PANCREATITIS IN CHILDHOOD

TRAUMA
INFECTIOUS
    Mumps
    Measles
    Rubella
    Coxsackie virus B
    Epstein-Barr virus
    Hepatitis A virus
    Influenza A virus
    Mycoplasma

OBSTRUCTIVE
- Annular pancreas
- Ascariasis
- Choledochocele
- Choledochal cyst
- Cholelithiasis
- Enteric duplication cyst
- Pancreatic pseudocyst
- Peptic ulcer disease
- Postoperative
- Duodenal stricture
- Tumor

DRUGS AND TOXINS
- Alcohol
- Azathioprine
- Corticosteroids
- Estrogens
- Furosemide
- L-Asparaginase
- Parenteral nutrition
- Scorpion bites
- Sulfasalazine
- Sulfonamides
- Tetracycline
- Thiazides
- Valproic acid

SYSTEMIC
- Crohn disease
- Cystic fibrosis
- Diabetes mellitus
- Hyperlipoproteinemia
  - Types I and IV
- Henoch-Schönlein purpura
- Hyperparathyroidism
- Malnutrition
- Periarteritis nodosa
- Peptic ulcer
- Sarcoidosis
- Systemic lupus erythematosus
- Uremia

Modified from: *Principles and Practice of Pediatrics*, Oski FA, DeAngelis CD, Feigin RD, Warshaw JB (eds), J.B. Lippincott Company, Philadelphia, 1990; p.1745.

Manual of Pediatric Gastroenterology, Fitzgerald JF, Clark JH (eds), Churchill Livingstone, New York City, 1988, p.91.

CAUSES OF HYPERAMYLASEMIA

PANCREATITIS
PANCREATIC PSEUDOCYST
PANCREATIC TRAUMA
PANCREATIC CARCINOMA
PAROTITIS
BILIARY TRACT DISEASE
DUODENAL ULCER
ISCHEMIC ENTEROCOLITIS
INTESTINAL OBSTRUCTION
ACUTE APPENDICITIS
PERITONITIS
RUPTURED ECTOPIC PREGNANCY
HEAD TRAUMA
BURNS
DIABETIC KETOACIDOSIS
UREMIA
POSTOPERATIVE
NEOPLASMS
    Pulmonary
    Ovarian
    Colonic
DRUGS

Modified from: *Textbook of Pediatric Gastroenterology*, Silverberg M, Daum F (eds), 2nd Edition, Year Book Medical Publishers, Inc., Chicago, 1988, p.385.

CAUSES OF GIANT SPLENOMEGALY

CHRONIC LEUKEMIAS
HAIRY CELL LEUKEMIA
LYMPHOMA
GAUCHER DISEASE
MALARIA
THALASSEMIA MAJOR
SARCOIDOSIS

Modified from: *Difficult Diagnosis in Pediatrics*, Stockman JA III (ed), W.B. Saunders Company, Philadelphia, 1990, p.308.

DISORDERS ASSOCIATED WITH HYPERSPLENISM

PRIMARY HYPERSPLENISM
SECONDARY HYPERSPLENISM
    Acute infections with splenomegaly
    Chronic infections
        Tuberculosis
        Brucellosis
        Malaria
        Kala-azar
    Inflammatory conditions
        Felty syndrome
        SLE
        Sarcoidosis
    Congestive splenomegaly
    Storage disorders
    Malignant disorders
    Chronic hemolytic disorders
    Myeloproliferative disorders
    Splenic malformations
    Hyperthyroidism
    Hypersplenism-Hypogammaglobulinemia
      syndrome

Modified from: *Difficult Diagnosis in Pediatrics*,
Stockman JA III (ed), W.B. Saunders Company, Philadelphia,
1990, p.309.

CAUSES OF ABDOMINAL MASS

BILIARY SYSTEM
    Choledochal cyst
    Hydrops of the gallbladder
HEPATOMEGALY
INTESTINAL
    Appendiceal abscess
    Crohn disease
    Duplication
    Fecal mass
    Intussusception
    Lymphoma
    Mesenteric cyst
    Perforation
    Volvulus
PANCREAS
    Pseudocyst
RETROPERITONEAL MASS
    Neuroblastoma
    Ganglioneuroma
    Adrenal cyst
    Sarcoma
RENAL ENLARGEMENT
    Wilm tumor
    Renal vein thrombosis
    Hydronephrosis
    Cystic kidney disease
SPLENOMEGALY
UTERUS, OVARY, VAGINA
    Pregnancy
    Hydrometrocolpos
    Pelvic inflammatory disease
    Rhabdomyosarcoma
    Ovarian cyst
    Teratoma
BLADDER DISTENSION

Modified from: *Practical Paediatric
Gastroenterology*, Walker-Smith JA, Hamilton JR,
Walker WA (eds), Butterworths, London, 1983, p.44.

DIFFERENTIAL DIAGNOSIS OF ASCITES

PORTAL HYPERTENSION
Portal vein thrombosis
Cirrhosis
Liver tumors
Budd-Chiari syndrome
Constrictive pericarditis
Congestive heart failure
HYPOALBUMINEMIA
Nephrotic syndrome
Protein-losing enteropathy
Malnutrition
PERITONITIS, INFECTIOUS
CHYLOUS
VENTRICULOPERITONEAL SHUNTS
PERITONEAL MALIGNANCY
PANCREATITIS

Modified from: *Principles and Practice of Pediatrics*
Oski FA, DeAngelis CD, Feigin RD, Warshaw JB (eds), J.B.
Lippincott Company, Philadelphia, 1990, p.1741.

COMMON CAUSES OF ABDOMINAL PAIN IN INFANCY

INTUSSUSCEPTION
HIRSCHSPRUNG ENTEROCOLITIS
STRANGULATED HERNIA
TRAUMA
MECKEL DIVERTICULITIS
BACTERIAL ENTEROCOLITIS
PNEUMONITIS
PYELONEPHRITIS
INTESTINAL OBSTRUCTION/VOLVULUS

Modified from: *Principles and Practice of Pediatrics*,
Oski FA, DeAngelis CD, Feigin RD, Warshaw JB (eds), J.B.
Lippincott Company, Philadelphia, 1990, pp.2023-2024.

Hatch EI: *Pediatric Clinics of North America* 32:1161,
1985.

DIFFERENTIAL DIAGNOSIS OF ACUTE PELVIC PAIN IN ADOLESCENT FEMALES

GYNECOLOGIC CAUSES
Dysmenorrhea
Endometriosis
Endometritis
Ectopic pregnancy
Hematocolpos
Mittelschmerz
Pelvic inflammatory disease
Rupture of ovarian cyst
Torsion of ovarian cyst
Septic abortion
Threatened abortion
Tubo-ovarian abscess
NONGYNECOLOGIC CAUSES
Appendicitis
Meckel diverticulitis
Gastroenteritis
Mesenteric adenitis
Intestinal obstruction
Inflammatory bowel disease
Cystitis
Pyelonephritis
Renal calculi

Modified from: Goldstein DP: *Pediatric Clinics of North America* 36:575, 1989.

COMMON CAUSES OF ABDOMINAL PAIN IN CHILDHOOD

APPENDICITIS
BACTERIAL ENTEROCOLITIS
VIRAL GASTROENTERITIS
PNEUMONIA
INFLAMMATORY BOWEL DISEASE
PYELONEPHRITIS
MECKEL DIVERTICULITIS
TRAUMA
INFECTIOUS MONONUCLEOSIS
DIETARY INDISCRETION

FOOD POISONING
PHARYNGITIS
DIABETES MELLITUS
HEPATITIS

Modified from: *Principles and Practice of Pediatrics*,
Oski FA, DeAngelis CD, Feigin RD, Warshaw JB (eds), J.B.
Lippincott Company, Philadelphia, 1990, pp.2044.

Hatch EI: *Pediatric Clinics of North America* 32:1161,
1985.

COMMON CAUSES OF CHRONIC DIARRHEA

INFECTIOUS DIARRHEA
POSTINFECTIOUS DIARRHEA
PSEUDOMEMBRANOUS COLITIS
ALLERGIC GASTROENTEROPATHY
CYSTIC FIBROSIS
IRRITABLE BOWEL SYNDROME
CELIAC DISEASE
INFLAMMATORY BOWEL DISEASE
SHORT BOWEL SYNDROME
HIRSCHSPRUNG DISEASE
MALROTATION
PARENTERAL INFECTIONS
PRIMARY CARBOHYDRATE MALABSORPTION

Modified from: *The Best of the Whole Pediatrician
Catalogs I-III*, McMillan JA, Stockman JA III, Oski FA
(eds), W.B. Saunders Company, Philadelphia, 1984, p.333

Gall DG, Hamilton JR: *Pediatric Clinics of North America*
21:1001-1017, 1974.

EXTRAINTESTINAL MANIFESTATIONS OF INFLAMMATORY BOWEL DISEASE

WEIGHT LOSS
GROWTH FAILURE
ARTHRITIS/ARTHRALGIAS
APHTHOUS STOMATITIS
ERYTHEMA NODOSUM
PYODERMA GANGRENOSUM
CONJUNCTIVITIS/IRITIS
CLUBBING OF FINGERS
CHRONIC ACTIVE HEPATITIS
PHLEBOTHROMBOSIS
ANEMIA
NEPHROLITHIASIS
PANCREATITIS
PERIANAL DISEASE

Modified from: *Textbook of Gastroenterology and Nutrition in Infancy*, Lebenthal E (ed), 2nd Edition, Raven Press, New York City, 1989, pp.1285-1286.

Textbook of Pediatric Gastroenterology, Silverberg M, Daum F (eds), Year Book Medical Publishers, Chicago, 1988, p.398.

CAUSES OF BLACK STOOL

MELENA
INGESTION OF IRON PREPARATIONS
INGESTION OF BISMUTH
INGESTION OF LEAD
INGESTION OF LICORICE
INGESTION OF CHARCOAL, COAL, OR DIRT

Modified from: *The Best of the Whole Pediatrician Catalogs I-III*, McMillan JA, Stockman JA III, Oski FA (eds), W.B. Saunders Company, Philadelphia, 1984, p.342.

CAUSES OF FALSE POSITIVE GUAIAC STOOL

INGESTION OF MEAT IN THE DIET WITHIN
    96 HOURS
INORGANIC IRON INGESTION

Modified from: *A Manual of Laboratory Diagnostic Tests*,
Fishbach FT (ed), 2nd Edition, J.B. Lippincott Company,
Philadelphia, 1987, p.196.

CAUSE OF FALSE NEGATIVE GUAIAC STOOL

INGESTION OF LARGE QUANTITIES OF VITAMIN C

Modified from: Jaffe RM, et al: *Annals of Internal
Medicine* 83:824-826, 1975.

CAUSES OF DILATED RECTUM

CHILD ABUSE
CONSTIPATION
HEMOLYTIC UREMIC SYNDROME
SUSTAINED DUODENAL TRAUMA

Modified from: Stockman JA III: *Journal Club Newsletter*
4:8, 1989.

ETIOLOGIES OF GI BLEEDING IN THE NEONATE

INGESTED MATERNAL BLOOD
REFLUX ESOPHAGITIS
GASTRITIS
STRESS ULCER
NECROTIZING ENTEROCOLITIS
PROTEIN-SENSITIVE ENTEROCOLITIS
MIDGUT VOLVULUS
COAGULOPATHY
HEMORRHAGIC DISEASE OF THE NEWBORN
VASCULAR MALFORMATIONS
HIRSCHSPRUNG ENTEROCOLITIS
INFECTIOUS ENTEROCOLITIS
ANAL FISSURE
GASTROINTESTINAL DUPLICATION CYST
IATROGENIC TRAUMA

Modified from: *Manual of Pediatric Gastroenterology*, Fitzgerald JF, Clark JH (eds), Churchill Livingstone, Inc., New York City, 1988, pp.109-110.

Oldham KT, Lobe TE: *Pediatric Clinics of North America* 32:1252-1253, 1985.

ETIOLOGIES OF GI BLEEDING IN INFANCY

ANAL FISSURE
ESOPHAGITIS
GASTRITIS
PEPTIC ULCER
INTUSSUSCEPTION
INFECTIOUS GASTROENTERITIS
PROTEIN-SENSITIVE ENTEROCOLITIS
MECKEL DIVERTICULUM
THROMBOCYTOPENIA
DRUG INGESTION (SALICYLATES, STEROIDS,
    CAUSTIC SUBSTANCES)
DUPLICATION CYSTS
VASCULAR MALFORMATIONS
VOLVULUS

Modified from: *Manual of Pediatric Gastroenterology*, Fitzgerald JF, Clark JH (eds), Churchill Livingstone, Inc., New York City, 1988, pp.109-110.

Oldham KT, Lobe TE: *Pediatric Clinics of North America* 32:1252-1253, 1985.

ETIOLOGIES OF GI BLEEDING IN CHILDHOOD

ANAL FISSURE
ESOPHAGITIS
GASTRITIS
PEPTIC ULCER DISEASE
INFECTIOUS GASTROENTERITIS
POLYPS
INFLAMMATORY BOWEL DISEASE
COAGULOPATHY
THROMBOCYTOPENIA
MECKEL DIVERTICULUM
HENOCH-SCHÖNLEIN PURPURA
HEMOLYTIC-UREMIC SYNDROME
HEMORRHOIDS
INTUSSUSCEPTION
MALLORY-WEISS TEAR
VASCULAR MALFORMATIONS
VOLVULUS
ENTERIC DUPLICATION

Modified from: *Manual of Pediatric Gastroenterology*,
Fitzgerald JF, Clark JH (eds), Churchill Livingstone, Inc.,
New York City, 1988, pp.109-110.

Oldham KT, Lobe TE: *Pediatric Clinics of North America*
32:1252-1253, 1985.

NONSURGICAL CAUSES OF GASTROINTESTINAL BLEEDING

HEMATOLOGIC DISORDERS
    Hemophilia
    Iron deficiency
    Thrombocytopenia
    Vitamin K deficiency
SYSTEMIC DISORDERS
    Henoch-Schönlein purpura
    Idiopathic pulmonary hemosiderosis
    Milk allergy
    Pseudoxanthoma elasticum
    Scurvy
    Shigellosis
    Turner syndrome
    Uremia
DRUGS OR TOXINS
    Aspirin
    Iron poisoning
    Potassium chloride tablets
    Steroids

Modified from: *The Whole Pediatrician Catalog: A Compendium of Clues to Diagnosis and Management*, McMillan JA, Nieburg PI, Oski FA (eds), W.B. Saunders Company, Philadelphia, 1977, p.290.

CAUSES OF FALSE POSITIVE SWEAT TEST

ADRENAL INSUFFICIENCY
ANOREXIA NERVOSA
ATOPIC DERMATITIS
AUTONOMIC DYSFUNCTION (SEGMENTAL HYPOHIDROSIS)
CELIAC DISEASE
DIABETES INSIPIDUS (NEPHROGENIC)
ECTODERMAL DYSPLASIA
FAMILIAL CHOLESTASIS
FUCOSIDOSIS
GLYCOGEN STORAGE DISEASE, TYPE 1
HYPOGAMMAGLOBULINEMIA
HYPOPARATHYROIDISM
HYPOTHYROIDISM

KLINEFELTER SYNDROME
MALNUTRITION
MUCOPOLYSACCHARIDOSES

Modified from: *Principles and Practice of Pediatrics*, Oski FA, DeAngelis CD, Feigin RD, Warshaw JB (eds), J.B. Lippincott Company, Philadelphia, 1990, pp.1368-1369.

CAUSES OF FALSE NEGATIVE SWEAT TEST

PERIPHERAL EDEMA
CONGESTIVE HEART FAILURE
EARLY AGE/INADEQUATE SAMPLE

Modified from: MacLean WC Jr, Tripp RW: *J Pediatr* 83:86, 1973.

CAUSES OF CONSTIPATION

DYSFUNCTIONAL TOILET TRAINING
EMOTIONAL DISTURBANCES
MENTAL RETARDATION
IMMOBILITY
COW'S MILK INGESTION
DRUGS
LOW DIETARY FIBER
FUNCTIONAL ILEUS
PAINFUL DEFECATION
MENINGOMYELOCELE
SPINAL CORD INJURY/TUMOR
STARVATION
INTESTINAL STENOSIS/ATRESIA
IMPERFORATE ANUS/ANAL STENOSIS
HYPOTHYROIDISM
HYPOKALEMIA
HYPERCALCEMIA
HIRSCHSPRUNG DISEASE
MECONIUM ILEUS
ANTERIORLY PLACED ANUS

Modified from: *Principles and Practice of Pediatrics*, Oski FA, DeAngelis CD, Feigin RD, Warshaw JB (eds), J.B. Lippincott Company, Philadelphia, 1990, p.1783.

Hatch TF: *Pediatric Clinics of North America* 35:265, 1988.

DRUGS/TOXINS THAT MAY CAUSE CONSTIPATION

    ANTACIDS
    ANTICHOLINERGICS
    ANTICONVULSANTS
    ARSENIC
    BARIUM SULFATE
    BISMUTH
    DIURETICS
    IRON
    LEAD
    MERCURY
    MUSCLE PARALYZERS
    OPIATES
    PHENOTHIAZINES

Modified from: *Textbook of Pediatric Gastroenterology*, Silverberg M, Daum F (eds), 2nd Edition, Year Book Medical Publishers, Chicago, 1988, p.185.

CAUSES OF RECTAL PROLAPSE

    CONSTIPATION
    DIARRHEA
    CYSTIC FIBROSIS
    EXSTROPHY OF BLADDER
    MALNUTRITION
    MENINGOMYELOCELE
    REPAIR OF IMPERFORATE ANUS

Modified from: *Swenson's Pediatric Surgery*, Raffensperger JG (ed), Appleton & Lange, Norwalk, 1990, p.241.

CHAPTER VI

GENETICS

FREQUENCY OF CHROMOSOMAL DISORDERS AMONG LIVE-BORN INFANTS

    TRISOMY 21 (DOWN SYNDROME)
        1 in 600
    TRISOMY 18
        1 in 5000
    TRISOMY 13
        1 in 15,000
    KLINEFELTER SYNDROME (47,XXY)
        1 in 700 males
    XYY SYNDROME (47, XXY)
        1 in 800 males
    TRIPLE-X SYNDROME (47, XXX)
        1 in 1000 females
    TURNER SYNDROME (45,X, 45X/46XX,
      45X/46XY iso CHROMOSOME Xq)
        1 in 1500 females
    FRAGILE X MENTAL RETARDATION
        1 in 2000 males
        1 in 3000 females

Modified from: *Introduction to Human Biochemical and Molecular Genetics*, Beaudet AL, Seriver CR, Sly WS, et al (eds), McGraw-Hill, Inc, New York, 1990, p.20.

FREQUENCY OF SOME COMMON MONOGENIC DISORDERS AMONG LIVE-BORN INFANTS

AUTOSOMAL DOMINANT
Familial hypercholesterolemia   - 1 in 500
Adult polycystic kidney disease   - 1 in 1250
Huntington chorea   - 1 in 2500
Hereditary spherocytosis   - 1 in 5000
von Willebrand disease   - 1 in 8000
Marfan syndrome   - 1 in 20,000
Achondroplasia   - 1 in 50,000

AUTOSOMAL RECESSIVE

Sickle cell anemia	– 1 in 655 (U.S. blacks)
Cystic fibrosis	– 1 in 2500 (Caucasians)
	– 1 in 17,000 (U.S. blacks)
Tay-Sachs disease	– 1 in 3000 (Ashkenazi Jews)
Alpha-antitrypsin ZZ genotype	– 1 in 3500
Phenylketonuria	– 1 in 12,000 (average)
Mucopolysaccharidoses (all types together)	– 1 in 25,000
Glycogen storage diseases (all types together)	– 1 in 50,000

X-LINKED

Duchenne muscular dystrophy	– 1 in 7000 males
Hemophilia A	– 1 in 10,000 males
Fragile X mental retardation	– 1 in 2000 males
	– 1 in 3000 females

Modified from: *Introduction to Human Biochemical and Molecular Genetics*, Beaudet AL, Scriver CR, Sly WS, et al (eds), McGraw-Hill, Inc, New York, 1990, p.21.

CHARACTERISTICS OF CANDIDATES FOR THE DIAGNOSIS OF METABOLIC DISEASE

FAMILY HISTORY OF SIBLING DYING EARLY
OVERWHELMING ILLNESS IN THE NEONATAL PERIOD
VOMITING, PYLORIC STENOSIS
ACUTE ACIDOSIS, ANION GAP
MASSIVE KETOSIS
DEEP COMA
SEIZURES, ESPECIALLY MYOCLONIC
HICCUPS, CHRONIC
UNUSUAL ODOR

Modified from: *Maternal Fetal Medicine: Principles and Practice*, Creasy RK, Resnick R (eds), W.B. Saunders Company, Philadelphia, 1989, p.62.

FREQUENCY OF SOME INBORN ERRORS OF METABOLISM FOR WHICH NEWBORN SCREENING IS AVAILABLE

CYSTIC FIBROSIS	- 1 IN 2500
CONGENITAL HYPO-THYROIDISM	- 1 IN 6000
CYSTINURIA	- 1 IN 7000
PHENYLKETONURIA	- 1 IN 12,000
HISTIDINEMIA	- 1 IN 17,000
IMINOGLYCINURIA	- 1 IN 20,000
HARTNUP DISORDER	- 1 IN 26,000
HYPERPROLINEMIA	- 1 IN 40,000
GALACTOSEMIA	- 1 IN 57,000
BIOTINIDASE DEFICIENCY	- 1 IN 60,000
ADENOSINE DEAMINASE DEFICIENCY	- <1 IN 100,000
MAPLE SYRUP URINE DISEASE	- 1 IN 200,000
HOMOCYSTINURIA	- 1 IN 200,000

Modified from: *Introduction to Human Biochemical and Molecular Genetics*, Beaudet AL, Seriver CR, Sly WS, et al (eds), McGraw-Hill, Inc, New York, 1990, p.43.

RISK FOR DEVELOPING DIABETES

	IDDM	NIDDM
GENERAL POPULATION	0.1-0.25%	2.5-5%
SIBLING OF DIABETIC	5-10%	10-15%
OFFSPRING OF DIABETIC	2-5%	10-15%

Modified from: *Pediatrics*, Rudolph AM, Hoffman JIE (eds), 18th Edition, Appleton & Lange, Norwalk, 1987, p.288.

SYNDROMES WITH HEARING LOSS

FREQUENT
CHARGE Association
Cockayne syndrome
Craniometaphyseal dysplasia
Facioauriculovertebral spectrum
Fetal iodine deficiency effects
Fetal methyl mercury effects
Fetal rubella effects
Frontometaphyseal dysplasia
Hunter syndrome
Hurler syndrome
Kartagener syndrome
Killian/Teschler-Nicola syndrome
Levy-Hollister syndrome
Maroteaux-Lamy Mucopolysaccharidosis
syndrome
Marshall syndrome
Melnick-Fraser syndrome
Mohr syndrome
Morquio syndrome
Multiple lentigines syndrome
Multiple synostosis syndrome
Nager syndrome
Oto-Palato-Digital syndrome, type I
Oto-Palato-Digital syndrome, type II
Sclerosteosis
Senter syndrome
Stickler syndrome
Treacher Collins syndrome
Trisomy 13 syndrome
Waardenburg syndrome
18q - syndrome
OCCASIONAL
Acrodysostosis
Baller-Gerold syndrome
Bardet-Biedl syndrome
Camurati-Engelmann syndrome
Carpenter syndrome
Cerebrocostomandibular
CHILD Syndrome
Cleft lip sequence
Cleidocranial dysostosis
Crouzon syndrome
de Lange syndrome
Diastrophic dysplasia

Dyskeratosis congenita syndrome
Ectrodactyly, ectodermal dysplasia,
  cleft lip-palate syndrome
Fanconi pancytopenia syndrome
Fetal trimethadione effects
Fibrodysplasia ossificans
  progressiva syndrome
Imperforate anus, hypotonia,
  prominent forehead
Frontonasal dysplasia sequence
Hay-Wells syndrome
Hurler-Scheie compound syndrome
Johanson-Blizzard syndrome
Klippel-Feil sequence
Langer-Giedion syndrome
McCune-Albright syndrome
Metaphyseal chondrodysplasia,
  Jansen type
Miller syndrome
Müllerian duct, renal and cervical
  vertebral defects
Noonan syndrome
Oculodentodigital syndrome
Osteogenesis imperfecta syndrome,
  type I
Progeria syndrome
Rieger syndrome
Robin sequence
Saethre-Chotzen syndrome
Scheie syndrome
Townes syndrome
Trisomy 8 syndrome
Weill-Marchesani syndrome
X O S (partial)
Turner syndrome (partial)

DIABETES: DIFFERENTIATING FEATURES OF IDDM AND NIDDM

IDDM (TYPE I)
    Clinical characteristics
        Thin habitus
        Ketosis prone
    Age onset
        Predominantly young (<40 year)
    Insulin level
        Low to absent

Treatment
 Insulin required for life
Family studies
 Increased prevalence of IDDM
Twin studies
 <50% concordance in monozygotic
  twins
Association with other autoimmune
 endocrine disease and antibodies
  Yes
Islet cell antibodies
 Yes
HLA association
 Yes
Further subtypes
 DR 3 associated
 DR 4 associated

NIDDM (TYPE II)
 Clinical characteristics
  Obese
  Ketosis less likely
 Age of onset
  Predominantly older (>40 yr)
 Insulin levels
  Variable
 Treatment
  Diet control or
  hypoglycemics may be sufficient
 Family studies
  Increased prevalence of NIDDM
 Twin studies
  Close to 100% concordance in
   monozygotic twins
 Association with other autoimmune
  endocrine disease and antibodies
   No
 Islet cell antibodies
  No
 HLA associations
  Maturity onset diabetes of the
   young
 Further subtypes
  Mutant insulins

Modified from: *Pediatrics*, Rudolph AM, Hoffman JIE
(eds), 18th Edition, Appleton & Lange, Norwalk, 1987, p.287.

PRIMARY METABOLIC DISORDERS WITH SIGNIFICANT SKELETAL DYSPLASIA

CALCIUM OR PHOSPHORUS
> Hypophosphatemic rickets
> Pseudodeficiency rickets
> Late rickets
> Idiopathic hypercalciuria
> Hypophosphatasia
> Pseudohypoparathyroidism

COMPLEX CARBOHYDRATES
> Mucopolysaccharidoses
> Mucolipidoses including sialidoses
> Mannosidosis, fucosidosis
> Generalized gangliosidoses

LIPIDS
> Niemann-Pick disease
> Gaucher disease

NUCLEIC ACIDS
> Adenosine deaminase deficiency
> Others

AMINO ACIDS
> Homocystinuria
> Others

METALS
> Menkes kinky hair syndrome
> (X-linked copper transport
> defect)

Modified from: *Pediatrics*, Rudolph AM, Hoffman JIE (eds), 18th Edition, Appleton & Lange, Norwalk, 1987, p.332.

SKELETAL DYSPLASIAS THAT PRODUCE RELATIVELY SHORT LIMBS IN INFANTS OR CHILDREN

CHONDRODYSPLASIA PUNCTATA (RHIZOMELIC, DOMINANT, X-LINKED, OTHER FORMS)
CAMPOMELIC DYSPLASIA (VARIOUS FORMS)
ACHONDROPLASIA
DIASTROPHIC DYSPLASIA
CHONDROECTODERMAL DYSPLASIA
ASPHYXIATING THORACIC DYSPLASIA
MESOMELIC DYSPLASIAS (VARIOUS FORMS)
ACROMESOMELIC DYSPLASIA (VARIOUS FORMS)

HYPOCHONDROPLASIA
DYSCHONDROSTEOSIS
METAPHYSEAL CHONDRODYSPLASIAS (VARIOUS FORMS)
MULTIPLE EPIPHYSEAL DYSPLASIAS (VARIOUS
    FORMS)
PSEUDOACHONDROPLASIA (VARIOUS FORMS)
TRICHORHINOPHALANGEAL SYNDROME
ACRODYSPLASIA WITH RETINITIS PIGMENTOSA
    AND NEPHROPATHY (SALDINO-MAINZER)

Modified from: *Pediatrics*, Rudolph AM, Hoffman JIE
(eds), 18th Edition, Appleton & Lange, Norwalk, 1987, p.332.

SKELETAL DYSPLASIAS WITH RELATIVELY SHORT TRUNK IN INFANCY AND CHILDHOOD

METATROPIC
KNIEST
SPONDYLOEPIPHYSEAL DYSPLASIA CONGENITA
SPONDYLOEPIPHYSEAL DYSPLASIA TARDA
SPONDYLOEPIPHYSEAL DYSPLASIAS
        Catel-Schwartz-Jampel
        Other varieties
DYSOSTEOSCLEROSIS
MUCOPOLYSACCHARIDOSES I, II, IV, VI
MUCOLIPIDOSIS II

Modified from: *Pediatrics*, Rudolph AM, Hoffman JIE
(eds), 18th Edition, Appleton & Lange, Norwalk, 1987, p.333.

INBORN ERRORS OF METABOLISM THAT MAY HAVE METABOLIC ACIDOSIS AS A MAJOR COMPONENT

AMINOACIDOPATHIES
- Maple syrup urine disease
- Isovaleric acidemia
- 3-Methylcrotonylglycinuria
- 3-Hydroxy-3-methylglutaric aciduria
- Alpha-methylacetoacetic aciduria
- Propionic acidemia
- Methylmalonic acidemia
- Pyroglutamic acidemia
- Alpha-ketoadipic aciduria
- Glutaric acidemia
- Multiple carboxylase deficiency
- Hawkinsinuria

ORGANIC ACIDEMIAS
- Multiple acyl-CoA dehydrogenase deficiency (glutaric acidemia type II)
- Ethylmalonic aciduria
- y-Hydroxybutyric aciduria

DEFECTS IN CARBOHYDRATE METABOLISM
- Diabetes mellitus
- Fructose-1,6-diphosphatase deficiency
- Succinyl-CoA transferase deficiency
- Glycogen storage disease, type 1
- Pyruvate carboxylase deficiency
- Pyruvate dehydrogenase complex deficiency

Modified from: *Nelson Textbook of Pediatrics*, Behrman RE, Vaughan VC (eds), 13th Edition, W.B. Saunders Company, Philadelphia, 1987, p.278

MUCOPOLYSACCHARIDOSES – INHERITANCE, URINARY MUCOPOLYSACCHARIDES AND ENZYME DEFECT

HURLER SYNDROME – AR, (ALPHA-L-IDURONIDASE)
    Dermatan sulfate
    Heparan sulfate
SCHEIE SYNDROME – AR, (ALPHA-L-IDURONIDASE)
    Dermatan sulfate
    Heparan sulfate
HURLER-SCHEIE SYNDROME – AR,
  (ALPHA-L-IDURONIDASE)
    Dermatan sulfate
    Heparan sulfate
HUNTER SYNDROME – X-LINKED, (IDURONATE
  SULFATASE)
    Dermatan sulfate
    Heparan sulfate
SANFILIPPO SYNDROME
    Type A – AR, (Heparan N-sulfatase)
        Heparan sulfate
    Type B – AR, (alpha-N-
      acetylglucosaminidase)
        Heparan sulfate
    Type C – AR, (N-acetyl transferase)
        Heparan sulfate
    Type D – AR, (alpha-N-
      acetylglucosaminide-6-sulfatase)
        Heparan sulfate

MAROTEAUX-LAMY SYNDROME - AR,
  (GALACTOSAMINE-4-SULFATASE)
     Dermatan sulfate
B-GLUCURONIDASE DEFICIENCY - AR,
  (B-GLUCURONIDASE)
     Dermatan sulfate
     Heparan sulfate
MORQUIO SYNDROME - AR, (GALACTOSE-6-
  SULFATASE)
     Keratan sulfate
MORQUIO SYNDROME TYPE B-AR,
  (B-GALACTOSIDASE)
     B-Galactosyl oligosaccharides
     Keratan sulfate

AR = Autosomal recessive

Modified from: *Pediatrics*, Rudolph AM, Hoffman JIE
(eds), 18th Edition, Appleton & Lange, Norwalk, 1987,
p.313.

Nelson Textbook of Pediatrics, Behrman RE, Vaughan
VC (Eds), 13th Edition, W.B. Saunders Company,
Philadelphia, 1987, p.324

HUMAN GENETIC DISORDERS POTENTIALLY TREATABLE BY GENE REPLACEMENT THERAPY

CYSTIC FIBROSIS
IMMUNE DEFICIENCY: DISORDERS OF
  BONE-MARROW-DERIVED CELLS
     Adenosine deaminase
     Purine nucleoside phosphorylase
     Chronic granulomatous disease
     Carbonic anhydrase II
        (osteopetrosis)
     Complement deficiencies (monocyte-
        macrophage function only)
HEMATOPOIETIC DISORDER
     Thalassemia
     Sickle cell disease
DEFICIENCY OF SERUM PROTEINS
     Hemophilia
     Alpha 1-antitrypsin deficiency
     C1 esterase inhibitor deficiency
        (hereditary angioneurotic edema)
     Complement deficiencies
        (circulating function)

INBORN ERRORS OF METABOLISM: PRIMARY
  HEPATIC FUNCTION
    Urea cycle deficiency
        Carbamyl phosphate synthetase
        Ornithine transcarbamylase
        Argininosuccinate synthetase
        Argininosuccinate lyase
        Arginase
    Organic acid disorders
        Propionyl CoA carboxylase
        Methylmalonyl CoA mutase
    Phenylketonuria (phenylalanine
      hydroxylase)
    Galactosemia
    Homocystinuria
    Maple syrup urine disease
STORAGE DISEASES
    Bone marrow
        Gaucher disease
          (glucocerebrosidase)
        Fabry disease (galactosidase)
    Other
        Glycogen storage diseases (i.e.,
          Pompe disease)
        Mucopolysaccharidosis
    Central nervous system disorders
        Lesch-Nyhan syndrome (hypoxanthine
          phosphoribosyltransferase)
        Tay-Sachs disease (hexosaminidase)
FAMILIAL HYPERCHOLESTEROLEMIA
ENDOCRINE DISORDERS
    Juvenile diabetes mellitus
    Hypopituitarism
    Hypoparathyroidism
IMMUNOLOGIC DISORDERS
    Vaccines
    Lymphokines
MUSCLE DISEASES
    Skeletal muscle
        Duchenne muscular dystrophy/
          Becker muscular dystrophy
    Cardiac muscle
        X-linked dilated cardiomyopathy
        Endocardial fibroelastosis

Modified from: *The Science and Practice of Pediatric
Cardiology*, Garson A Jr, Bricker JT, McNamara DG (eds),
Lea & Febiger, Philadelphia, 1990, p.59.

Introduction to Human Biochemical & Molecular Genetics,
Beaudet AL, Scriver CR, Sly WS, et al (eds); McGraw Hill,
Inc, New York, 1990, p.49.

RISK FACTORS FOR ATHEROSCLEROSIS AND CORONARY ARTERY DISEASE

LDL RECEPTOR GENOTYPE
APOLIPROPROTEIN E GENOTYPE
FAMILIAL HYPERTRIGLYCERIDEMIA
FAMILIAL COMBINED HYPERLIPIDEMIA
LIPOPROTEIN Lp(a)
INCREASED LDL
DECREASED HDL
AGING
MALE SEX
SMOKING
HYPERTENSION
OBESITY
DIET
DIABETES MELLITUS
INACTIVITY
STRESS

Modified from: *Introduction to Human Biochemical & Molecular Genetics*, Beaudet AL, Scriver CR, Sly WS, et al (eds), McGraw Hill, Inc, New York, 1990, p.49.

INCIDENCE OF MINOR ANOMALIES AND NORMAL VARIATIONS IN NEWBORN INFANTS

PHYSICAL FEATURE	WHITE INFANTS (%) (N=3989)	BLACK INFANTS (%) (N=827)
Third sagittal fontanel	3.1	9.8
Epicanthal folds, bilateral	1.4	1.0
Brushfield spots, bilateral	7.2	0.2
Preauricular sinus, left or right	0.8	5.3
Extra nipple, left or right	0.5	4.6
Umbilical hernia	0.7	6.1
Sacral dimple	4.8	0.6
Clinodactyly of both 5th fingers	5.2	4.5
Simian crease, both hands	0.7	0.5
Syndactyly of toes 2 & 3, left or right	1.7	2.3

Modified from: *Nelson Textbook of Pediatrics*, Behrman RE, Vaughan VC (eds), 13th Edition, W.B. Saunders Company, Philadelphia, 1987, p.268

SELECTED DISORDERS AND RESPECTIVE GENE LOCI LOCATION

DISORDER	LOCATION
Acute alcohol intolerance	12q24.2
Acute lymphoblastic leukemia	9p22–p21
Adrenal hyperplasia, congenital, due to 11-beta-hydroxylase deficiency	8q21
Adrenal hyperplasia, congenital, due to 21-hydroxylase deficiency	6p21.3
Adrenal hyperplasia II	1p13
Adrenal hyperplasia V	Chr.10
Adrenal hyperplasia primary	Xp21.3–p21.2
AFP deficiency, congenital	4q11–q13
Agammaglobulinemia, type 2, X-linked	Xp22
Agammaglobulinemia, X-linked	Xq21.3–q22
Alport syndrome	Xq22–q24
Alzheimer disease	21q11.2–q21
Antithrombin III deficiency	1q23.1–q23.9
Ataxia-telangiectasia	11q22–q23
Atrial septal defect, secundum type	6p21.3
Becker muscular dystrophy	Xp21.2
Beckwith-Wiedemann syndrome	11pter–p15.4
Burkett lymphoma	8q24.1
Chronic granulomatous disease due to deficiency of NCF-1	Chr.7
Chronic granulomatous disease due to deficiency of NCF-2	1cen–q32
Cleft palate, X-linked	Xq21
Craniosynostosis	7p21.3–p21.2
Cystic fibrosis	7q31.3–q32
Diabetes insipidus, nephrogenic	Xq28
?Diabetes insipidus, neurohypophyseal 125700	Chr.20
?Diabetes mellitus, insulin dependent	6p21.3
Diabetes mellitus, insulin-resistant, with acanthosis nigricans	19p13.3–p13.2
DiGeorge syndrome	22q11
Duchenne muscular dystrophy	Xp21.2
Ehlers-Danlos syndrome, type IV	2q31
Ehlers-Danlos syndrome, type VIIA1	17q21.31–q22.05
Ehlers-Danlos syndrome, type VIIA2	7q21.3–q22.1
Ehlers-Danlos syndrome, type X	2q34–q36

DISORDER	LOCATION
Ewing sarcoma	22q12
Fabry disease	Xq22
Factor V deficiency	1q23
Factor VII deficiency	13q34
Factor X deficiency	13q34
Factor XI deficiency	4q35
Factor XII deficiency	5q33-qter
Factor XIII, A component deficiency	6p25-p24
Favism	Xq28
Friedreich ataxia	9q13-q21.1
Fructose intolerance	9q22
Fucosidosis	1p34
G6PD deficiency	Xq28
Galactokinase deficiency	17q21-q22
Galactosemia	9p13
Gaucher disease	1q21
Glycogen storage disease, type VII	1cen-q32
Glycogen storage disease VIII	Xq12-q13
GM1-gangliosidosis	3p21-p14.2
GM2-gangliosidosis, AB variant	Chr.5
GM2-gangliosidosis, juvenile, adult	15q22-q25.1
Gonadal dysgenesis, XY female type	Xp22-p21
Granulomatous disease, chronic, X-linked	Xp21.1
?Growth hormone deficiency, X-linked	Xq21.3-q22
?Gynecomastia, familial, due to increased aromatase activity	15q21.1
Hemochromatosis	6p21.3
Hemolytic anemia due to G6PD deficiency	Xq28
Hemolytic anemia due to PGK deficiency	Xq13
Hemophilia A	Xq28
Hemophilia B	Xq27.1-q27.2
Huntington disease	4p16.3
Hurler syndrome	22q11
Hydrops fetalis	19cen-q12
Hypercholesterolemia, familial	19p13.2-p13.1
Hypothyroidism, nongoitrous	1p22

DISORDER	LOCATION
Hypothyroidism, nongoitrous, due to TSH resistance	22q11-q13
Immunodeficiency, X-linked, with hyper-IgM	Xq24-q27
Incontinentia pigmenti	Xp11.2
Incontinentia pigmenti, familial	Xq27-q28
Interferon, alpha, deficiency	9p21
?Isolated growth hormone deficiency due to defect in GHRF	20p11.23-qter
Isolated growth hormone deficiency IIIig type with absent GH and Kowarski type with bioinactive GH	17q22-q24
?Kostmann agranulocytosis	6p21.3
Krabbe disease	Chr.17
?Lactase deficiency, adult, 223100	Chr.2
?Lactase deficiency, congenital	Chr.2
?Letterer-Siwe disease	13q14-q31
?Leukemia, acute lymphocytic, with 4/11 translocation	4q21
Leukemia, acute T-cell	11p13
Leukemia, T-cell acute lymphocytic	10q24
Leukemia/lymphoma, B-cell,1	11q13.3
Leukemia/lymphoma, B-cell,2	18q21.3
Leukemia/lymphoma, T-cell	14q32.1
Leukemia/lymphoma, T-cell	14q11.2
Maple syrup disease	Chr.19
Marfan syndrome, atypical	7q21.3-q22.1
Menkes disease	Xq12-q13
Mucopolysaccharidosis I	22q11
Mucopolysaccharidosis II	Xq27.3
Mucopolysaccharidosis IVB	3p21-p14.2
Mucopolysaccharidosis VII	7q21.1-q22
Neuroblastoma	1p32
Neurofibromatosis, von Recklinghausen	17q11.2
Niemann-Pick disease	Chr.17
Omithine transcarbamylase deficiency	Xp21.1
Osteogenesis imperfecta, 2 or more clinical forms	7q21.31-q22.05
Osteogenesis imperfecta, 2 or more clinical forms	7q21.3-q22.1
Osteosarcoma, retinoblastoma-related	13q14.1
Phenylketonuria	12q24.1
Phenylketonuria due to dihydropteridine reductase deficiency	4p15.3
PK deficiency hemolytic anemia	1q21-q22

DISORDER	LOCATION
Polycystic kidney disease	16p13.31-p13.12
Pompe disease	17q23
Prader-Willi syndrome	15q11
Protein C deficiency	2q13-q14
Protein S deficiency	3p11.1-q11.2
Renal tubular acidosis-osteopetrosis syndrome	8q22
Retinoblastoma	13q14.1-q14.2
Rhabdomyosarcoma	11pter-p15.5
Rhabdomyosarcoma, aveolar	2q37
Rh-null disease	3cen-q22
?Rh-null hemolytic anemia	1p36.2-p34
Rieger syndrome	4q23-q27
Schizophrenia	5q11.2-q13.3
Severe combined immuno-deficiency due to ADA deficiency	20q13.11
Severe combined immunodeficiency (SCID), HLA class II-negative type	19p13
Sickle cell anemia	11p15.5
Sucrose intolerance	3q25-q26
Tay-Sachs disease	15q22-q25.1
Thalassemias, alpha-	16pter-p13.3
Thalassemias, beta-	11p15.5
?Treacher Collins mandibulofacial dysostosis	5q11
Trypsinogen deficiency	7q22-qter
Tuberous sclerosis-1	9q33-q34
Tuberous sclerosis-2	11q23
Vitamin D dependency, type I	12q14
(Vivax malaria, susceptibility to)	1q21-q22
von Willebrand disease	12pter-p12
Wilms tumor	11p13
Wilms tumor, type 2	11p15.5
Wilson disease	13q14-q21
Wiskott-Aldrich syndrome	Xp11.3-p11
Zellweger syndrome	7q11.12-q11.23

Modified from: *Introduction to Human Biochemical and Molecular Genetics*, Beaudet AL, Seriver CR, Sly WS, et al (eds), McGraw-Hill, Inc, New York, 1990, pp.121-133.

CHAPTER VII

GENITOURINARY TRACT

CAUSES OF FALSE POSITIVE PROTEIN BY DIPSTICK

LEACHING OF CITRATE BUFFER
  Overlong immersion in urine
  Holding strip in a urine stream
ALKALINE URINARY pH
QUATERNARY AMMONIUM COMPOUNDS USED TO
  CLEAN URINE RECEPTACLES
PYURIA
BACTERIURIA
MUCOPROTEIN

Modified from: *The Whole Pediatrician's Catalog*,
McMillan JA, Stockman JA, Oski FA (eds), W.B. Saunders
Company, Philadelphia, 1979, p.251.

CAUSES OF FALSE NEGATIVE PROTEIN BY DIPSTICK

INCOMPLETE WETTING OF STRIP
EXTREMELY LOW pH OF URINE
VERY DILUTE URINE

Modified from: *The Whole Pediatrician's Catalog*,
McMillan JA, Stockman JA, Oski FA (eds), W.B. Saunders
Company, Philadelphia, 1979, p.251.

CAUSES OF FALSE POSITIVE GLUCOSE BY DIPSTICK

BLEACH IN THE COLLECTING VESSEL
VAGINAL POWDERS CONTAINING GLUCOSE

Modified from: *The Whole Pediatrician's Catalog*,
McMillan JA, Stockman JA, Oski FA (eds), W.B. Saunders
Company, Philadelphia, 1979, p.249.

CAUSES OF FALSE POSITIVE DIPSTICK FOR HEMOGLOBIN

AGE OR CONDITION OF DIPSTICK
BACTERIAL PEROXIDASES
DELAY BETWEEN DIPSTICK AND SEDIMENT
    MICROSCOPY
HYPOCHLORITE CLEANSING SOLUTIONS
MYOGLOBINURIA
PROVIDONE IODINE SOLUTION

Modified from: Baker MD, Baldassano RN: *Pediatr Emerg Care* 5:241, 1989.

CAUSES OF FALSE POSITIVE URINE CLINITEST FOR GLUCOSE

GALACTOSE
LACTOSE
LEVULOSE
MALTOSE
PENTOSE
HEMOGENTISIC ACID
GLUCURONIC ACID
BLEACH
DRUGS
        Acetanalide
        P-aminosalicylic acid
        Antipyrine
        Cephaloridine
        Cephalothin
        Chloramphenicol
        Chlortetracycline
        Cinchophen
        Diatrizoate
        Isoniazid
        Levodopa
        Nalidixic acid
        Oxytetracycline
        Tetracycline

Modified from: *The Whole Pediatrician's Catalog*, McMillan JA, Stockman JA, Oski FA (eds), W.B. Saunders Company, Philadelphia, 1979, p.249.

CAUSES OF BROWN-BLACK URINE

HEMOGLOBIN
HOMOGENTISIC ACID
MELANIN
METHEMOGLOBIN
METHOCARBAMOL
METHYLDOPA
METRONIDAZOLE
NITRITES
NITROFURANS
PHENACETIN
PROVIDONE IODINE
RHUBARB
SENNA (ALKALINE URINE)
TYROSINOSIS (ALKALINE URINE)

Modified from: Baker MD, Baldassan RN: *Pediatr Emerg Care* 5:241, 1989.

CAUSES OF PINK/RED URINE

FOODS
    Beet pigment
    Blackberries
    Vegetable dyes
DRUGS
    Diphenylhydantoin
    Desferoxamine
    Methyldopa
    Phenindione
    Phenothiazine
    Phenolphthalein
    Pyridium
    Senna
HEMOGLOBINURIA
MYOGLOBINURIA
URATES
BLOOD
INFECTIONS
    Serratia

Modified from: *Clinical Paediatric Nephrology*, Postlethwaite RJ (ed), IOP Publishing Ltd, Bristol, 1986, p.27.

Baker MD, Baldassan RN: *Pediatr Emerg Care* 5:241, 1989.

CAUSES OF BLUE URINE

BILIVERDIN
INDIGO BLUE
METHYLENE BLUE
TRIAMTERINE

Modified from: Baker MD, Baldassan RN: *Pediatr Emerg Care* 5:241, 1989.

CAUSES OF ORANGE URINE

BILE
CONGO RED
RIFAMPIN
WARFARIN

Modified from: Baker MD, Baldassan RN: *Pediatr Emerg Care* 5:241,1989.

AMINO ACID DISORDERS ASSOCIATED WITH
URINE ODORS

Isovaleric acidemia	Sweaty feet
Glutaric acidemia	Sweaty feet
Maple syrup urine disease	Maple syrup
Methionine malabsorption	Cabbage
Phenylketonuria	Mousy
Trimethylaminuria	Rotting fish
Tyrosinemia	Rancid

Modified from: *Clinical Diagnosis and Management by Laboratory Methods*, Henry JB (ed), 17th Edition, W.B. Saunders Company, Philadelphia, 1984, p.392.

CAUSES OF GROSS HEMATURIA

INFECTION
STONES
TRAUMA
FOREIGN BODIES
TUMOR
CONGENITAL ABNORMALITIES
GLOMERULONEPHRITIS
BERGER DISEASE (IgA NEPHROPATHY)
BENIGN RECURRENT HEMATURIA
EXERCISE HEMATURIA
HEMOLYTIC UREMIC SYNDROME
SICKLE CELL TRAIT OR DISEASE
COAGULOPATHY
RENAL VENOUS THROMBOSIS
RENAL HEMANGIOMAS
DRUGS

Modified from: *Nephrology & Urology for the Pediatrician*, Gauthier B, Edelmann CM, Barnett ML (eds), Little, Brown and Company, Boston, 1982, p.94.

DRUGS AND CHEMICALS WHICH MAY CAUSE HEMATURIA

ANTICOAGULANTS
ANTIBACTERIALS
    Ampicillin
    Kanamycin
    Methicillin
    Penicillin
    Polymyxin
    Sulfonamides
MISCELLANEOUS DRUGS
    Aspirin
    Amitriptyline
    Benzotropine mesylate
    Chlorpromazine
    Colchicine
    Cyclophosphamide
    Indomethacin
    Phenylbutazone
    Trifluoperazine

SOLVENTS
    Carbon tetrachloride
    Phenol
    Turpentine
METALS
    Copper sulphate
    Lead
    Gold
    Phosphorous

Modified from: *Clinical Paediatric Nephrology*,
Postlethwaite RJ (ed), IOP Publishing Ltd, Bristol, 1986,
p.313.

CAUSES OF LACTIC ACIDOSIS

LESS THAN 5 MEQ/L
    Alkalosis
    Carbohydrate infusion
    Exercise
    Catecholamines
    Diabetic ketosis
    Alcohol
MORE THAN 5 MEQ/L
    Shock
    Severe anemia
    Hypoxia
    Glycogenoses
    Malignancies
    Phenformin
    Idiopathic

Modified from: Emmett M, Narins R: *Medicine* 56:38-54,
1977.

CAUSES OF DISTAL RENAL TUBULAR ACIDOSIS

FAMILIAL
MARFAN SYNDROME
EHLER-DANLOS SYNDROME
CARBONIC ANHYDRASE DEFICIENCY
WILSON DISEASE
ELLIPTOCYTOSIS
SICKLE CELL ANEMIA
HEREDITARY FRUCTOSE INTOLERANCE
AMYLOIDOSIS
MEDULLARY SPONGE KIDNEY
IDIOPATHIC HYPERCALCIURIA
HYPERPARATHYROIDISM
HYPERVITAMINOSIS D
HYPERTHYROIDISM
SJOGREN'S SYNDROME
HYPERGAMMAGLOBULINEMIA
RENAL TRANSPLANT REJECTION
MULTIPLE MYELOMA
SYSTEMIC LUPUS ERYTHEMATOSUS
AMPHOTERICIN B
LITHIUM CARBONATE
CYCLAMATES
ANALGESICS
TOLUENE
HEPATIC CIRRHOSIS

Modified from: *Difficult Diagnosis in Pediatrics*;
Stockman JA III (ed), W.B. Saunders Company,
Philadelphia, 1990, p.409.

**CAUSES OF A NORMAL ANION GAP METABOLIC
ACIDOSIS (HYPERCHLOREMIC ACIDOSIS)**

GASTROINTESTINAL BICARBONATE LOSS OR
  ORGANIC
  ACID ANIONS
      Diarrhea
      Pancreatic fistula
RENAL
      Uremic acidosis (early)
      Renal tubular acidosis
            Gradient - distal
            Bicarbonate wasting - proximal
            Aldosterone deficiency
URETEROSIGMOIDOSTOMY
DILUTIONAL ACIDOSIS
      Rapid I.V. hydration

HYPERALIMENTATION
ACIDOSIS AFTER RESPIRATORY ALKALOSIS
    (Post-hypocapnia)
DRUGS
    Carbonic anhydrase inhibitor
        Acetazolamide (Diamox)
        Mafenide (Sulfamylon)
    Anion exchange resin
        Cholestyramine
    Acidifying agents
        NH_4Cl
        $CaCl_2$
        Arginine HCl
        Lysine HCl

Modified from: Oh M, Carroll H: *N Engl J Med*
297:814-817, 1977.

Emmett M, Narins R: *Medicine* 56:38-54, 1977.

**CAUSES OF METABOLIC ACIDOSIS WITH
INCREASED ANION GAP (NORMOCHLOREMIC
ACIDOSIS)**

    KETOACIDOSIS
    LACTIC ACIDOSIS
    UREMIC ACIDOSIS
    HYPEROSMOLAR HYPERGLYCEMIC NONKETOTIC
      COMA
    INGESTION OF TOXINS
        Salicylate
        Methanol
        Ethylene glycol
        Paraldehyde

Modified from: Oh M, Carroll H: *N Engl J Med*
297:814-817, 1977.

CAUSES OF METABOLIC ALKALOSIS

CHLORIDE-RESPONSIVE
- Pyloric stenosis
- Vomiting
- Nasogastric drainage
- Congenital chloride diarrhea
- Diuretic therapy
- Poorly reabsorbable anion therapy (carbenicillin, penicillin)
- Posthypercapnia
- Chloride-deficient formulas
- Cystic fibrosis
- Exogenous alkali
- Contraction alkalosis

CHLORIDE-RESISTANT
- Hyperreninism
- Primary hyperaldosteronism
- Cushing syndrome
- Bartter syndrome
- Excessive intake of licorice
- Severe potassium depletion
- Hypercalcemia
- Hyperparathyroidism
- Magnesium deficiency
- Adrenal enzyme deficiency
- Liddle syndrome
- Chewing tobacco

Modified from: *Critical Care Clinics* 3:699-955, 1987.

CAUSES OF INCREASED ANION GAP

DECREASED UNMEASURED CATION
     Hypokalemia
     Hypocalcemia
     Hypomagnesemia
INCREASED UNMEASURED ANION
     Organic anions
          Lactate
          Ketone acids
     Inorganic anions
          Phosphate
          Sulfate
     Proteins
          Hyperalbuminemia (transient
            after albumin infusion)
     Exogenous anions
          Salicylate ingestion
          Ethylene glycol ingestion
          Methanol ingestion
          Paraldehyde ingestion
          Penicillin
          Carbenicillin
          Hyperosmolar hyperglycemic
           nonketotic coma
          Formate
          Nitrate
     Laboratory error
          Falsely increased serum sodium
          Falsely decreased serum
           chloride or bicarbonate

Modified from: Oh M, Carroll H: *N Engl J Med* 297:814-817, 1977.

CAUSES OF DECREASED ANION GAP

INCREASED UNMEASURED CATION
      Increased concentration of normally
        present cation
            Hyperkalemia
            Hypercalcemia
            Hypermagnesemia
      Retention of abnormal cation
            IgG globulin
            Lithium
DECREASED UNMEASURED ANION
      Hypoalbuminemia
LABORATORY ERROR
      Falsely decreased serum sodium
            Viscous serum
            Hyperglycemia
            Hyperlipidemia
            Random error
      Falsely increased serum chloride
            Bromide intoxication
      Falsely increased serum bicarbonate

Modified from: Oh M, Carroll H: *N Engl J Med*
297:814-817, 1977.

CAUSES OF FANCONI SYNDROME

PRIMARY
      Hereditary
      Sporadic
SECONDARY
      Cystinosis
      Galactosemia
      Fructose intolerance
      Lowe syndrome
      Glycogen storage disease
        (glu-6-phosphatase deficiency)
      Tyrosinemia
      Wilson disease
      Nephrotic syndrome
      Multiple myeloma
      Renal transplant rejection

Heavy metal intoxication
Outdated tetracycline ingestion
Sjögren syndrome
Renal vein thrombosis
Vitamin D deficiency rickets

Modified from: *Difficult Diagnosis in Pediatrics*,
Stockman JA III (ed), W.B. Saunders Company, Philadelphia,
1990, p.409.

Clinical Paediatric Nephrology, Postlethwaite RJ (ed),
IOP Publishing Ltd, Bristol, 1986, p.244.

CAUSES OF HYPERKALEMIA

PSEUDOHYPERKALEMIA
Leukocytosis
Thrombocytosis
Hemolysis (in vitro)
Improper collection or handling of
blood
INCREASED POTASSIUM LOAD
Oral potassium supplementation
Intravenous administration
Salt substitutes
Potassium penicillin in high doses
Potassium pooling in intravenous
bags
Stored blood
Endogenous cell breakdown
Trauma
Intravascular hemolysis
Burns
Rhabdomyolysis
Major surgery
Total starvation
Chemotherapy of lymphomas,
leukemia, myeloma
DECREASED RENAL POTASSIUM EXCRETION
Acute oliguric renal failure
Chronic renal failure
Adrenal insufficiency
Hypoaldosteronism
18-OH dehydrogenase defect
21-hydroxylase defect
Hyporeninemic hypoaldosteronism

Drugs
        Succinylcholine
        Arginine hydrochloride
        Digitalis poisoning
Defective tubular secretion
        Sickle cell disease
        Systemic lupus erythematosus
        Renal transplantation (acute)
        Obstructive uropathy
        Interstitial nephritis
        Spitzer-Weinstein syndrome
        Low birth weight infants
Potassium sparing diuretics
        Triamterene
        Spironolactone
REDISTRIBUTION
        Acidosis (metabolic or respiratory)
        Severe exercise with beta blockade
          (propranolol)
        Increased ECF osmolality (glucose,
          mannitol, saline)
        Hyperkalemic periodic paralysis

Modified from: *Pediatric Nephrology*, Holliday MA,
Barratt TM, Vernier RL (eds), 2nd Edition, Williams &
Wilkins, Baltimore, 1987, p.21.

CAUSES OF HYPOKALEMIA

DECREASED INTAKE
        Inadequate K^+ in diet or IV fluid
        Ingestion of K^+ binding clay
INCREASED INTRACELLULAR K^+ UPTAKE
        Alkalosis
        Hyperinsulinism
        Increased beta adrenergic agonist
          activity
        Pseudohypokalemia
        Early in the course of treatment of
          megaloblastic anemia
        Transfusion with frozen washed RBC
        Intravenous hyperalimentation
        Periodic hypokalemic paralysis
        Hypothermia
        Barium chloride ingestion

INCREASED GASTROINTESTINAL K⁺ LOSS
    Vomiting
    Diarrhea
        Infectious
        Laxative abuse
    Intestinal fistula, tube drainage
    Ureterosigmoidostomy
    Villous adenoma of colon (adults)
    Overuse of K⁺ binding resins
INCREASED LOSS THROUGH EXCESSIVE
    SWEATING
OVER ZEALOUS DIALYSIS AGAINST A LOW K⁺
    BATH
INCREASED K⁺ LOSS FROM KIDNEY
    Drugs
        Diuretics
        Antibiotics
            Amphotericin
            Carbenicillin
            Gentamicin
            Clindamycin
            Rifampin
            Out-dated tetracycline
            Polymycin B
            Ampicillin
            Penicillin
        Corticosteroids
        Levodopa
        Cisplatin
POLYURIA
OSMOTIC DIURESIS
    Glucose
    Mannitol
HYPERCALCEMIA
HYPOMAGNESEMIA
ACID BASE DISORDERS
    Metabolic alkalosis with
        bicarbonate loss
    Metabolic acidosis with bicarbonate
        loss
    RTA type 1- deficient H+ secretion
    RTA type 2- bicarbonate wasting
    Organic anions - Diabetic
        ketoacidosis

RENAL SALT WASTING WITH PRIMARY RENAL
   DISEASES
      RTA
      Bartter syndrome
      Fanconi syndrome
      Pyelonephritis
      Obstructive uropathy
      Acute leukemia
EXCESSIVE PRIMARY MINERALOCORTICOID
   ACTIVITY WITH LOW PLASMA RENIN
      Primary hyperaldosteronism
      Adrenogenital syndrome
         17-alpha-hydroxylase
            deficiency
         11-beta-hydroxylase deficiency
      Cushing syndrome
EXCESSIVE SECONDARY MINERALOCORTICOID
   ACTIVITY WITH HIGH RENIN
      Malignant hypertension
      Renal artery stenosis
      Renin producing tumor
      Necrotizing vasculitis
STATES OF PSEUDOHYPERALDOSTERONISM
      Liddle syndrome
      Licorice abuse
      Carbonoxolone
      Fludrocortisone

Modified from: Linshaw MA: *Pediatric Clinics of North
America* 34:661, 1987.

DISORDERS ASSOCIATED WITH HYPERCALCIURIA

TYPE I RENAL TUBULAR ACIDOSIS
IMMOBILIZATION
HIGH DIETARY CALCIUM
SARCOIDOSIS
DIURETIC THERAPY
   Furosemide
SYNDROME OF INAPPROPRIATE ADH SECRETION
HYPERPARATHYROIDISM
CUSHING SYNDROME
CORTICOSTEROID THERAPY
MEDULLARY SPONGE KIDNEY

```
LEAD POISONING
TUBULAR DYSFUNCTION
        Fanconi syndrome
        Wilson disease
JUVENILE RHEUMATOID ARTHRITIS
```

Modified from: Heiliczer JD, Canonigo BB, Bishof NA, Moore ES: *Pediatric Clinics of North America* 34:713, 1987.

DISORDERS ASSOCIATED WITH UROLITHIASIS

```
CALCIUM LITHIASIS
        Hypercalciuric states
                Idiopathic hypercalciuria
                Distal renal tubular acidosis
                Drug-induced (furosemide)
                Primary hyperparathyroidism
                Immobilization
                Hyperthyroidism
                Adrenocorticosteroid excess
                Adrenal insufficiency
                Osteolytic metastases
                Hypervitaminosis D
                Idiopathic hypercalcemia of
                    infancy
                Sarcoidosis
                Milk-alkali syndrome
HYPEROXALURIA
        Hereditary hyperoxaluria
        Enteric hyperoxaluria
        Associated with pyridoxine
            deficiency
        Idiopathic calcium urolithiasis
            (adult)
HYPERURICOSURIA
HYPOCITRATURIA
        Distal renal tubular acidosis
        Gastrointestinal disease
URIC ACID LITHIASIS
STRUVITE LITHIASIS
        Infections
CYSTINURIA
```

INBORN ERRORS OF METABOLISM
        Hereditary xanthinuria
        Orotic aciduria
GENITOURINARY TRACT ANOMALIES

Modified from: *Clinical Paediatric Nephrology*,
Postlethwaite RJ (ed), IOP Publishing Ltd, Bristol,
1986, p.399.

CAUSES OF INAPPROPRIATE SECRETION OF ANTIDIURETIC HORMONE

CNS
        Infection
        Tumor
        Injury
        Vascular accidents
        Guillain-Barré syndrome
POSTSURGERY
        Anesthetic or premedication
        Cardiac bypass surgery
        Peritoneal reflexes
        Intracranial manipulation
INFECTION
        Acute infectious diseases
            (especially viral)
PULMONARY
        Asthma
        Infection
        Emphysema
        Fibrosis
        Tumors
        Ventilation
CARDIAC
        Cardiac bypass surgery
        Cardiac failure
        Constrictive pericarditis
DRUG RELATED
METABOLIC
        Acute intermittent porphyria

Modified from: *Clinical Paediatric Nephrology*,
Postlethwaite RJ (ed), IOP Publishing Ltd, Bristol,
1986, p.22.

CAUSES OF RENAL CONCENTRATING DEFECT

FANCONI SYNDROME
OSMOTIC DIURETICS
COMPULSIVE WATER DRINKING
DRUGS
     Lithium
     Demeclocycline
     Propoxyphene
     Methoxyflurane
ELECTROLYTE DISORDERS
     Hypercalcemia
     Hypokalemia
SYSTEMIC DISORDERS
     Sickle cell disease
     Amyloidosis
     Sjögren syndrome
RENAL PARENCHYMAL DISEASE
     Chronic renal failure
     Obstructive nephropathy
     Medullary cystic disease
     Polycystic kidney disease
     Interstitial nephritis
ACUTE RENAL FAILURE

Modified from: *Clinical Paediatric Nephrology*,
Postlethwaite RJ (ed), IOP Publishing Ltd, Bristol, 1986,
p.248.

MAJOR CAUSES OF ACUTE NEPHRITIS

LOW SERUM COMPLEMENT LEVEL
     Systemic diseases
          Systemic lupus erythematosus
          Subacute bacterial
            endocarditis
          "Shunt" nephritis
          Cryoglobulinemia
     Renal diseases
          Acute poststreptococcal
            glomerulonephritis
          Membranoproliferative
            glomerulonephritis

NORMAL SERUM COMPLEMENT LEVEL
Systemic diseases
Polyarteritis nodosa
Hypersensitivity vasculitis
Wegener granulomatosis
Henoch-Schönlein purpura
Goodpasture syndrome
Visceral abscess
Renal diseases
IgG-IgA nephropathy
Idiopathic rapidly progressive
glomerulonephritis
Anti-glomerular basement
membrane disease
Immune-complex disease
Negative immunofluorescence
findings

Modified from: Madaio M, Harrington J: *N Engl J
Med* 309:1299-1302, 1983.

INFECTIOUS AGENTS ASSOCIATED WITH
   ACUTE NEPHRITIS

STREPTOCOCCUS - GROUP A BETA-HEMOLYTIC
STAPHYLOCOCCUS
PNEUMOCOCCUS
KLEBSIELLA
MENINGOCOCCUS
SALMONELLA
MYCOPLASMA PNEUMONIAE
COXSACKIE VIRUS
ECHOVIRUS
EPSTEIN-BARR VIRUS
HEPATITIS B VIRUS
INFLUENZA VIRUS
MUMPS VIRUS
RUBEOLA VIRUS

Modified from: *Clinical Paediatric Nephrology*,
Postlethwaite RJ (ed), IOP Publishing Ltd, Bristol,
1986, p.164.

CAUSES OF RHABDOMYOLYSIS

IDIOPATHIC
DIRECT MUSCLE INJURY
    Trauma
    Burns
EXCESSIVE MUSCULAR ACTIVITY
    Sports
    Seizures
    Delirium tremens
    Status asthmaticus
    Psychosis
ISCHEMIA
    Compression
    Vascular occlusion
    Sickle cell trait
    Air embolism
GENETIC DISORDERS
    Abnormal carbohydrate metabolism
    Abnormal lipid metabolism
    Muscular dystrophies
METABOLIC DISORDERS
    Diabetes mellitus
    Hypokalemia
    Hyponatremia
    Hypernatremia
    Hypophosphatemia
    Myxedema
IMMUNOLOGIC
    Dermatomyositis
    Polymyositis
INFECTIONS
    Tetanus
    Legionnaire disease
    Influenza
    Infectious mononucleosis
    Bacterial pyomyositis
DRUGS
    Heroin
    Methadone
    Phencyclidine
    Amphetamines
    LSD
    Glutethimide
    Salicylate overdose
    Succinylcholine
    Clofibrate
    Epsilon aminocaproic acid

TOXINS
    Ethanol
    Isopropyl alcohol
    Carbon monoxide
    Mercuric chloride
    Ethylene glycol
    Toluene
    Snake bites
    Hornet or wasp sting
    Brown spider bite

Modified from: *The Kidney*, Brenner BM, Rector FC Jr
(eds), 3rd Edition, W.B. Saunders Company,
Philadelphia, 1986, p.745.

CAUSES OF PYURIA WITHOUT BACTERIURIA

DEHYDRATION
TRAUMA
PRESENCE OF AN IRRITANT IN THE RENAL
    PELVIS, BLADDER OR URETER
RENAL TUBERCULOSIS
ACUTE AND CHRONIC GLOMERULONEPHRITIS
AFTER ADMINISTRATION OF ORAL POLIO
    VACCINE
AFTER ADMINISTRATION OF INTRAMUSCULAR
    IRON
RENAL TUBULAR ACIDOSIS
IN ASSOCIATION WITH A VARIETY OF VIRAL
    INFECTIONS
KAWASAKI SYNDROME

Modified from: *The Whole Pediatrician's Catalog*,
McMillan JA, Stockman JA, Oski FA (eds), W.B. Saunders
Company, Philadelphia, 1979, p.251.

CAUSES OF TRANSIENT HYPERTENSION

ACUTE GLOMERULONEPHRITIS
HEMOLYTIC UREMIC SYNDROME
HENOCH-SCHÖNLEIN NEPHRITIS
ACUTE RENAL FAILURE
FOLLOWING UROLOGICAL SURGERY
FOLLOWING RENAL TRANSPLANTATION
ACUTE HYPOVOLEMIA
CENTRAL NERVOUS SYSTEM DISEASE
    Tumor
    Infection
    Injury
    Seizures
GUILLAIN-BARRE SYNDROME
POLIOMYELITIS
FAMILIAL DYSAUTONOMIA
HYPERCALCEMIA
LEAD POISONING
DRUG THERAPY OR OVERDOSE
    Corticosteroids
    Sympathomimetics
    Oral contraceptives
HYPERVOLEMIA DUE TO EXCESS
  ADMINISTRATION OF:
    Blood
    Plasma
    Saline
IMMOBILIZATION

Modified from: *Pediatric Nephrology*, Holliday MA,
Barratt TM, Vernier RL (eds), 2nd Edition, Williams &
Wilkins, Baltimore, 1987, p.750.

CAUSES OF SUSTAINED HYPERTENSION IN CHILDHOOD

COARCTATION OF AORTA
RENOVASCULAR DISEASE
     Renal artery stenosis
     Renal artery aneurysm
     Arteriovenous fistula
     Renal artery thrombosis
     Polyarteritis nodosa
RENAL PARENCHYMAL DISEASE
     Coarse renal scarring
     Chronic glomerulonephritis
     Polycystic kidneys
     Renal dysplasia
     Hemolytic uremic syndrome
RENAL TUMORS
PHEOCHROMOCYTOMA
NEUROBLASTOMA
CONGENITAL ADRENAL HYPERPLASIA
CONN AND CUSHING SYNDROME
ESSENTIAL HYPERTENSION
DRUG USE

Modified from: *Clinical Paediatric Nephrology*, Postlethwaite RJ (ed), IOP Publishing Ltd, Bristol, 1986, p.5.

ETIOLOGIES OF ASYMPTOMATIC PROTEINURIA

BENIGN
     Transient or functional
     Orthostatic
     Persistent
GLOMERULAR
     Glomerulonephritis
     Minimal change disease
TUBULO-INTERSTITIAL
     Interstitial nephritis
     Primary tubular disorders
     Renal hypoplasia/dysplasia
     Pyelonephritis
     Reflux nephropathy
OVERLOAD
     Monoclonal gammopathies
     Leukemia

Modified from: *Difficult Diagnosis in Pediatrics*, Stockman JA III (ed), W.B. Saunders Company, Philadelphia, 1990, p.328.

CLINICAL CONDITIONS ASSOCIATED WITH EDEMA IN INFANCY

PHYSIOLOGICAL
CARDIAC
RENAL
HYPOXIA IN UTERO
HYALINE MEMBRANE DISEASE
ERYTHROBLASTOSIS FETALIS
LYMPHEDEMA
CONGENITAL ASCITES
METABOLIC
    Vitamin E deficiency
    Hypomagnesemia and hypocalcemia
    Cystic fibrosis
TURNER SYNDROME

Modified from: *Clinical Paediatric Nephrology*,
Postlethwaite RJ (ed), IOP Publishing Ltd, Bristol, 1986,
p.8.

CLINICAL CONDITIONS ASSOCIATED WITH GENERALIZED EDEMA IN CHILDREN

NEPHROTIC SYNDROME
ACUTE GLOMERULONEPHRITIS
ACUTE RENAL FAILURE
CHRONIC RENAL FAILURE
CONGESTIVE HEART FAILURE
HEPATIC FIBROSIS
HEPATIC VENOUS OUTFLOW OBSTRUCTION
VENA CAVAL OBSTRUCTION
HYPOTHYROIDISM
CAPILLARY LEAK SYNDROME

Modified from: *Clinical Paediatric Nephrology*,
Postlethwaite RJ (ed), IOP Publishing Ltd, Bristol, 1986,
p.67.

CAUSES OF ACUTE SCROTAL PAIN

INCARCERATED HERNIA
TORSION OF THE TESTIS
TORSION OF THE APPENDIX TESTIS
ACUTE HYDROCELE
INGUINAL LYMPHADENITIS
ACUTE EPIDIDYMITIS
ACUTE ORCHITIS
BLUNT TRAUMA
TRAUMATIC HEMATOCELE OR HYDROCELE
SCROTAL CELLULITIS

Modified from: Nakayama DK, Rowe MI: *Pediatrics in Review* 11:87-93, 1989.

Signs and Symptoms in Pediatrics, Tunnessen WW (ed), 2nd Edition, J.B. Lippincott Company, Philadelphia, 1988, pp.462-464.

CHAPTER VIII

GROWTH AND DEVELOPMENT

CAUSES OF TALL STATURE

CONSTITUTIONAL TALL STATURE
DIABETES MELLITUS (EARLY)
EXCESS ANABOLIC STEROID
    Adrenal tumor
    Congenital adrenal hyperplasia
    Gonadal hormones or gonadotropin-
       secreting tumors
    Precocious puberty
    Premature adrenarche or pubarche
EXCESS GROWTH HORMONE
    Pituitary tumor
HYPERTHYROIDISM
MISCELLANEOUS
    Cerebral gigantism
    Hereditary abnormalities of the
      skeleton
    Homocystinuria
    Hypogonadism in the male
        Kallmann syndrome
        Klinefelter syndrome
    Marfan syndrome
    Neurofibromatosis
    Polyostotic fibrous dysplasia
      (Albright syndrome)
    Testicular feminization syndrome
      (pubertal)

Modified from: Maurice D, Kogut MD: *Pediatric Clinics of North America* 20:801, 1973.

SECONDARY CAUSES OF OBESITY

ACQUIRED HYPOTHALAMIC LESIONS
ALSTROM SYNDROME
BLOUNT SYNDROME
CARPENTER SYNDROME
COHEN SYNDROME
CUSHING SYNDROME
DOWN SYNDROME
HYPOTHYROIDISM
LAURENCE-MOON-BIEDL SYNDROME
PRADER-WILLI SYNDROME
PRIMARY HYPERINSULINISM
     Beckwith-Wiedemann syndrome
     Insulinoma
     Nesidioblastosis
STEIN-LEVENTHAL SYNDROME

Modified from: Rosenbaum M, Leibel RL: *Pediatrics in Review* 11:52, 1989.

CONDITIONS ASSOCIATED WITH DELAYED CLOSURE OF THE ANTERIOR FONTANEL

ACHONDROPLASIA
AMINOPTERIN EMBRYOPATHY
APERT SYNDROME
CLEIDOCRANIAL DYSOSTOSIS
CONGENITAL RUBELLA
DOWN SYNDROME
FETAL HYDANTOIN EFFECTS
HALLERMANN-STREIFF SYNDROME
HYPOPHOSPHATASIA
HYPOTHYROIDISM
INCREASED INTRACRANIAL PRESSURE
KENNY SYNDROME
MALNUTRITION
OSTEOGENESIS IMPERFECTA
PROGERIA

PYKNODYSOSTOSIS
RICKETS
RUSSELL-SILVER SYNDROME
ZELLWEGER SYNDROME

Modified from: *Pediatric Neurology Principles and Practice*, Swaiman KF (ed), C.V. Mosby Company, St. Louis, 1989, p.345.

The Whole Pediatrician's Catalog: A Compendium of Clues to Diagnosis and Management, McMillan JA, Nieburg PI, Oski FA (eds), W.B. Saunders Company, Philadelphia, 1977, p.4.

CONDITIONS ASSOCIATED WITH EARLY CLOSURE OF THE ANTERIOR FONTANEL

MICROCEPHALY
HIGH Ca^{++}/VITAMIN D RATIO IN PREGNANCY
CRANIOSYNOSTOSIS
HYPERTHYROIDISM
NORMAL VARIANT

Modified from: *The Whole Pediatrician's Catalog: A Compendium of Clues to Diagnosis and Management*, McMillan JA, Nieburg PI, Oski FA (eds), W.B. Saunders Company, Philadelphia, 1977, p.4.

CAUSES OF DELAYED DENTITION

AARSKOG SYNDROME
ALBRIGHT HEREDITARY OSTEODYSTROPHY
CHONDROECTODERMAL DYSPLASIA
CLEIDOCRANIAL DYSOSTOSIS
CORNELIA DE LANGE SYNDROME
DUBOWITZ SYNDROME
FETAL RUBELLA
FRONTO-METAPHYSEAL DYSPLASIA
GARDNER SYNDROME
GOLTZ SYNDROME
HUNTER SYNDROME
INCONTINENTIA PIGMENTI SYNDROME
KILLIAN/TESCHLER-NICOLA SYNDROME
MAROTEAUX-LAMY MUCOPOLYSACCHARIDOSIS
    SYNDROME
MILLER-DIEKER SYNDROME
OSTEOGENESIS IMPERFECTA SYNDROME, TYPE 1
PROGERIA SYNDROME
X-LINKED HYPOPHOSPHATEMIC RICKETS

Modified from: *Smith's Recognizable Patterns of Human Malformation*, Jones KL (ed), 4th Edition, W.B. Saunders Company, Philadelphia, 1988, p.731.

SIGNS AND SYMPTOMS OF TEETHING

DAYTIME RESTLESSNESS
INCREASE IN FINGER SUCKING
GUM RUBBING
DROOLING
LOSS OF APPETITE, POSSIBLY

Modified from: *The Whole Pediatrician's Catalog*, McMillan JA, Stockman JA III, Oski FA (eds), W.B. Saunders Company, Philadelphia, 1979, p.73.

ORGANIC CAUSES OF ACUTE CRYING DURING INFANCY

GENERAL
- Drug ingestion or overdosage
- Pruritic or painful rash

EYES
- Corneal abrasion

EAR, NOSE, THROAT
- Otitis media
- Pharyngitis
- Mouth ulcers
- Stuffy nose

CARDIOVASCULAR
- Congestive heart failure
- Supraventricular tachycardia
- Acute hypertension

GENITOURINARY
- Urinary tract obstruction or infection
- Meatal ulcer
- Torsion of testis or ovary

GASTROINTESTINAL
- Acute abdomen
- Acute constipation
- Anal fissures
- Gastroenteritis
- Ingested foreign body
- Inguinal hernia
- Intussusception
- Reflux esophagitis
- Volvulus
- Colic

NEUROLOGIC
- Increased intracranial pressure

SKELETAL
- Arthritis
- Fracture
- Hair or thread twisted around digit
- Sickle cell vasoocclusive crisis
- Scurvy
- Subperiosteal hematoma

Modified from: *Difficult Diagnosis in Pediatrics*, Stockman JA III (ed), W.B. Saunders Company, Philadelphia, 1990, p.184.

CHAPTER IX

HEMATOLOGY

CAUSES OF NEONATAL ANEMIA

SECONDARY TO BONE MARROW SUPPRESSION OR BLOOD LOSS
Congenital hypoplastic anemia
Drug-induced red cell suppression
Internal hemorrhage
Fetomaternal hemorrhage
Fetoplacental hemorrhage
Twin-twin transfusion
Umbilical cord rupture or hematoma
Placental trapping

SECONDARY TO HEMOLYSIS
ABO hemolytic disease
Rh hemolytic disease
Minor blood group incompatibilities
Disseminated intravascular coagulopathy
Mechanical red cell destruction
Infections: viral, bacterial, toxoplasmosis, and malaria
Phenolic disinfectant
Vitamin E deficiency
Drug induced hemolysis
Maternal autoimmune hemolytic anemia
Membrane defects
Enzyme defects
Hemoglobinopathies (usually after several months)
Others: osteopetrosis, galactosidase deficiency, hypothyroidism

CAUSES OF LOW MCV

COMMON
Iron deficiency
Thalassemia trait
Alpha
Beta

LESS COMMON
Lead poisoning
Chronic disease
Protein calorie malnutrition
Copper deficiency
Sideroblastic anemia

CAUSES OF ELEVATED MCV

    NORMAL NEWBORN
    RETICULOCYTOSIS
    SPURIOUS ELEVATIONS (Cold Agglutinins)
    HYPOTHYROIDISM
    LIVER DYSFUNCTION
    DOWN SYNDROME
    HEREDITARY OROTIC ACIDURIA
    B_{12}/FOLATE DEFICIENCY
    APLASTIC ANEMIA
    PRELEUKEMIA
    LEUKEMIA
    DIAMOND-BLACKFAN SYNDROME

CAUSES OF INCREASED FREE ERYTHROCYTE (ZINC) PROTOPORPHYRIN

    LEAD POISONING
    IRON DEFICIENCY
    CHRONIC DISEASE
    NORMAL NEWBORNS
    ERYTHROPOIETIC PROTOPORPHYRIA
    ERYTHROPOIETIC COPROPORPHYRIA
    CONGENITAL ERYTHROPOIETIC PORPHYRIA
    SIDEROBLASTIC ANEMIA
    SECONDARY POLYCYTHEMIAS

CAUSES OF NUCLEATED RBC'S

    NORMAL NEWBORN (first 3-5 days)
    ACUTE HYPOXIC EVENT
    ACUTE BLEEDING
    SEVERE HEMOLYTIC ANEMIA
    CONGENITAL INFECTIONS
    POSTSPLENECTOMY OR HYPOSPLENIC STATES
    DYSERYTHROPOIETIC ANEMIAS
    MEGALOBLASTIC ANEMIA
    LEUKOERYTHROBLASTIC REACTIONS

CAUSES OF HOWELL-JOLLY BODIES

ASPLENIC AND HYPOSPLENIC STATES
PERNICIOUS ANEMIA
SEVERE IRON DEFICIENCY ANEMIA
DYSERYTHROPOIETIC ANEMIA

CAUSES OF BASOPHILIC STIPPLING

THALASSEMIA
LEAD POISONING
IRON DEFICIENCY
UNSTABLE HEMOGLOBINS
PYRIMIDINE 5' NUCLEOTIDASE DEFICIENCY

CAUSES OF TEARDROP CELLS

NORMAL NEWBORN
THALASSEMIA MAJOR
LEUKOERYTHROBLASTIC REACTION
MYELOPROLIFERATIVE SYNDROME

CAUSES OF SPHEROCYTES

HEREDITARY SPHEROCYTOSIS
ABO INCOMPATIBILITY
AUTOIMMUNE HEMOLYTIC ANEMIA
MICROANGIOPATHIC HEMOLYTIC ANEMIA
SICKLE CELL DISEASE
HYPERSPLENISM
BURNS
POST-TRANSFUSION
PYRUVATE KINASE DEFICIENCY
WATER DILUTION HEMOLYSIS
SEVERE HYPOPHOSPHATEMIA WITH HEMOLYSIS
CLOSTRIDIAL SEPSIS
SPIDER, BEE AND SNAKE VENOMS
HEMOLYTIC TRANSFUSION REACTION
ACUTE OXIDANT INJURY

CAUSES OF TARGET CELLS

    THALASSEMIA SYNDROMES
    IRON DEFICIENCY
    HEMOGLOBIN S, C, D, and E
    OBSTRUCTIVE LIVER DISEASE
    FAMILIAL LECITHIN: CHOLESTEROL
       ACYLTRANSFERASE DEFICIENCY (LCAT)
    POST-SPLENECTOMY

AGENTS ASSOCIATED WITH THE DEVELOPMENT
OF APLASTIC ANEMIA

    DRUGS
              Acetazolamide
              Amodiaquine
              Arsenicals
              Barbiturates
              Chloramphenical
              Chlordiazepoxide
              Colchicine
              Gold
              Hydantoins
              Indandiones
              Meprobamate
              Methicillin
              Oxazolidones
              Phenothiazines
              Potassium perchlorate
              Pyrazolones (phenylbutazone)
              Pyrimethamine
              Quinacrine
              Quinidine, quinine
              Ristocetin
              Stibophen
              Streptomycin
              Sulfamyl compounds
              Sulfonamides
              Sulfonylureas
              Thiazides
              Thiocarbamates
              Thiocyanate
              Thiosemicarbazones
              Thiouracils
              Tripelennamine
    TOXINS

INSECTICIDES
Chlordane
Chlorophenothane (DDT)
Gamma benzene hexachloride
(Lindane)
Parathione
SOLVENTS
Benzene
Carbon tetrachloride
Glue
Stoddard's solvent
Toluene
Trinitrotoluene
RADIATION

Modified from: *Hematology of Infancy and Childhood*, Nathan DG, Oski FA (eds), 3rd Edition, W.B. Saunders Company, Philadelphia, 1987, p.161.

INFECTIOUS CAUSES OF APLASTIC ANEMIA

PARVOVIRUS
EBV (infectious mononucleosis)
HEPATITIS Non-A, Non-B
HEPATITIS B
HEPATITIS A

Modified from: *Hematology of Infancy and Childhood*, Nathan DG, Oski FA (eds), 3rd Edition, W.B. Saunders Company, Philadelphia, 1987, p. 161.

PRELEUKEMIC BONE MARROW FAILURE SYNDROMES

ACQUIRED
Aplastic anemia
Radiation
Drugs
Toxins
Pure red cell aplasia
Paroxysmal nocturnal hemoglobinuria
Refractory sideroblastic anemia
Pre-acute lymphocytic leukemia
Myelodysplastic syndromes
Myeloproliferative disorders

CONSTITUTIONAL
    Fanconi anemia
    Kostmann agranulocytosis
    Shwachman-Diamond neutropenia
    Diamond-Blackfan anemia
    Amegakaryocytic thrombocytopenia
    Familial marrow failure
    Familial myeloproliferative disease
    Trisomy 21
    Bloom syndrome
    Ataxia-telangiectasia
    Poland syndrome

Modified from: *Hematology of Infancy and Childhood*,
Nathan DG, Oski FA (eds), 3rd Edition, W.B. Saunders
Company, Philadelphia, 1987, pp.215-219.

AGENTS COMMONLY PRODUCING HEMOLYSIS IN PATIENTS WITH G6PD DEFICIENCY

    METHYLENE BLUE
    NALIDIXIC ACID
    NAPHTHALENE (moth balls)
    CHLOROQUINE
    NITROFURANTOIN
    PRIMAQUINE
    PAMAQUINE
    DIPHENYLSULFONE
    SULFANILAMIDE
    SULFACETAMIDE
    SULFAPYRIDINE
    SULFISOXAZOLE
    CHLORAMPHENICOL
    QUINACRINE
    BENZENE
    FAVISM (fava bean)
    ASCORBIC ACID
    ACETYLSALICYLIC ACID

Modified from: *Hematology of Infancy and Childhood*,
Nathan DG, Oski FA (eds), 3rd Edition, W.B. Saunders
Company, Philadelphia, 1987, p.599.

CAUSES OF POLYCYTHEMIAS

PRIMARY
> Polycythemia vera
> Familial polycythemia

SECONDARY
> Cardiac disease with left to right shunting
> Pulmonary disease
> High altitude
> Pickwickian syndrome
> High oxygen affinity hemoglobinopathy
> Carboxyhemoglobin
> Methemoglobin
> Low cardiac output
> Decreased red cell 2,3 DPG
> Decreased tissue oxygen utilization
> Wilms tumor
> Cerebellar hemangioblastoma
> Hepatoma
> Renal cell carcinoma
> Uterine leiomyomas
> Ovarian carcinoma
> Renal cysts
> Hydronephrosis
> Bartter syndrome
> Adrenocorticoid excess
> Testosterone administration
> Growth hormone administration
> Pheochromocytoma

RELATIVE
> Dehydration
> Spurious (stress or smokers') erythrocytosis

Modified from: *Hematology of Infancy and Childhood*
Nathan DG, Oski FA (eds), 3rd Edition, W.B. Saunders
Company, Philadelphia, 1987, p.1070.

POLYCYTHEMIA IN THE NEONATE

INTRAUTERINE HYPOXIA OR INFECTION
PLACENTAL DYSFUNCTION
- Dysmaturity
- Postmaturity

DEVELOPMENTAL DEFECTS IN NEONATES
- Small for gestational age
- Down syndrome
- Infant of a diabetic mother
- Adrenal hyperplasia
- Oligohydramnios
- Trisomy D

TRANSFUSIONS
- Twin-twin
- Maternal-fetal
- Placenta-cord

HEMATOLOGIC ABNORMALITIES ASSOCIATED WITH DOWN SYNDROME

MACROCYTOSIS
ELEVATED RETICULOCYTE COUNT
NEONATAL POLYCYTHEMIA
CONGENITAL THROMBOCYTOPENIA
INCREASED INCIDENCE OF ERYTHROBLASTOSIS
LEUKEMIA
MYELOPROLIFERATIVE DISORDER
PLATELET BIOCHEMICAL ALTERATION
ELEVATED PLASMA VISCOSITY

Modified from: *Down's Anomaly*, Smith GF, Berg JM (eds), Churchill Livingstone, 1976, pp.100-118.

CAUSES OF ACQUIRED SPLENIC HYPOFUNCTION AND ATROPHY

ADULT CELIAC DISEASE AND SPRUE
DERMATITIS HERPETIFORMIS
FANCONI ANEMIA
HEMOGLOBIN S DISORDERS
THOROTRAST ADMINISTRATION
THYROTOXICOSIS
ULCERATIVE COLITIS

Modified from: *Hematology of Infancy and Childhood*, Nathan DG, Oski FA (eds), 3rd Edition, W.B. Saunders Company, Philadelphia, 1987, p.905.

INFECTIONS ASSOCIATED WITH NEUTROPENIA

BACTERIAL
- Typhoid fever
- Paratyphoid fever
- Tuberculosis (disseminated)
- Brucellosis
- Gram-negative sepsis

VIRAL
- Infectious hepatitis
- Infectious mononucleosis
- Influenza
- Measles
- Rubella
- Roseola
- Varicella
- Dengue fever
- Colorado tick fever
- Smallpox
- Poliomyelitis
- Yellow fever
- Sand-fly fever
- Psittacosis
- Mumps
- Cytomegalovirus
- Lymphocytic choriomeningitis virus

RICKETTSIAL
- Rocky Mountain spotted fever
- Typhus fever
- Rickettsial pox

FUNGAL
- Histoplasmosis

PROTOZOAL
- Malaria
- Leishmaniasis (Kala-azar)

Modified from: Weetman RM, Boxer LA: *Pediatric Clinics of North America* 27(2):361-375, 1980.

DRUGS ASSOCIATED WITH NEUTROPENIA

ANTIBACTERIAL DRUGS
- Carbenicillin
- Cephalosporins
- Chloramphenicol
- Penicillins
- Sulfonamides
- Vancomycin

ANTIPHLOGISTIC DRUGS
- Aminopyrine
- Phenylbutazone
- Dipyrone

ANTITHYROID AND ANTIRHEUMATIC DRUGS
- Propylthiourasil
- Gold thiomalate

TRANQUILIZING DRUGS
- Chlorpromazine
- Meprobamate
- Mepazine
- Promazine hydrochloride

CYTOTOXIC AGENTS
- Cyclophosphamide
- Methotrexate
- 6-Thioguanine
- Cytosine arabinoside
- Adriamycin

Modified from: Weetman RM, Boxer LA: *Pediatric Clinics of North America* 27(2):361-375, 1980.

DISORDERS ASSOCIATED WITH NEUTROPHIL DYSFUNCTION

MARGINATION AND ADHERENCE
- Posthemodialysis
- Endotoxic shock
- Pancreatitis

CHEMOTATIC DISORDERS
- A variety of dermatitis conditions
- Job syndrome - hyper IgE and IgA
- Acquired during infection
- Actin dysfunction
- Hyperalimentation and malnutrition
- Diabetes
- Shwachman-Diamond syndrome
- Normal newborn infant
- Complement deficiencies and dysfunction
- Serum inhibitors
  - IgA
  - Lymphokines
  - Immune complexes
  - Complement inactivation

RECOGNITION AND INGESTION
- Impaired opsonization
  - Immunoglobulin deficiency
  - Complement deficiency
  - Newborn infant
  - Sickle cell disease
- Actin dysfunction
- Defective granule function
  - Chediak-Higashi syndrome
- Defective peroxidative killing
  - Chronic granulomatous disease
  - Glucose-6-phosphate dehydrogenase deficiency
  - Myeloperoxidase deficiency
  - Auto-oxidative defects
    - Glutathione reductase deficiency
    - Glutathione synthetase deficiency
    - Vitamin E deficiency states

Modified from: Baehner RL: *Pediatric Clinics of North America* 27(2):385, 1980.

CAUSES OF LEUKOCYTOSIS

PHYSIOLOGIC
    Normal newborn (maximal 38,000/mm^3)
    Strenuous exercise
    Emotional disorders - fear, agitation
    Ovulation
        Labor
        Pregnancy

ACUTE INFECTIONS
    Bacterial
    Viral
    Fungal
    Protozoal
    Spirochetal

METABOLIC CAUSES
    Diabetic coma
    Acidosis
    Anoxia
    Azotemia
    Thyroid storm
    Acute gout
    Burns
    Seizures

MALIGNANT NEOPLASMS
    Carcinoma
    Sarcoma
    Lymphoma

ACUTE HEMORRHAGE

DRUGS
    Steroids
    Epinephrine
    Endotoxin
    Lithium
    Serotonin
    Histamine
    Heparin
    Acetylcholine

TOXINS
    Lead
    Mercury
    Camphor

CONNECTIVE TISSUE DISEASES
    Rheumatic fever
    Rheumatoid arthritis
    Inflammatory bowel disease

HEMATOLOGIC DISEASES
        Splenectomy
        Functional asplenia
        Leukemia
        Myeloproliferative disorders
        Hemolytic anemia
        Transfusion reaction
        Infectious mononucleosis
        Megaloblastic anemia during therapy
        Postagranulocytosis

Modified from: *Manual of Pediatric Hematology and Oncology*, Lanzkowsky P (ed), Churchill Livingstone, New York, 1989, p.132.

CAUSES OF LYMPHOCYTOSIS

INFECTION
        Pertussis
        Infectious mononucleosis
        Infectious lymphocytosis
        Infectious hepatitis
        Cytomegalovirus
        Toxoplasmosis
        Syphilis
        Brucellosis
        Common viral illnesses
HEMATOLOGIC
        Lymphocytic leukemias
        Neutropenias
MISCELLANEOUS
        Thyrotoxicosis
        Addison disease

Modified from: *Hematology of Infancy and Childhood*, Nathan DG, Oski FA (eds), W.B. Saunders Company, Philadelphia, 1987, p.1665.

CAUSES OF LYMPHOCYTOPENIA

    INFECTION
        Active tuberculosis
        Malaria
    COLLAGEN VASCULAR DISEASE
        Systemic lupus erythematosus
        Regional enteritis
    CERTAIN IMMUNODEFICIENCY SYNDROMES
    ENDOCRINE DISORDERS
        Hyperadrenalism
        Adrenal corticosteroid administration
    HEMATOLOGIC AND ONCOLOGIC
        Hodgkin disease
        Solid tumors
        Aplastic anemia
    EXCESSIVE LOSSES
        Thoracic duct drainage
        Intestinal lymphangiectasias

Modified from: *Hematology of Infancy and Childhood*,
Nathan DG, Oski FA (eds), W.B. Saunders Company,
Philadelphia, 1987, p.1665.

CAUSES OF EOSINOPHILIA

    ALLERGIC
        Asthma
        Hay fever
        Chronic rhinitis
            Drug reaction
            Atopic dermatitis
            Urticaria
        PARASITES
            Pneumocystis carinii infection
            Hookworms
            Scabies
            Amebiasis
            Toxoplasmosis
            Ascariasis
            Visceral larva migrans
            Trichinosis

NEOPLASMS
     Brain tumors
     Hodgkin and non-Hodgkin lymphomas
HEMATOLOGIC DISORDERS
     Fanconi anemia
     Thrombocytopenia with absent radius
     Chronic myeloproliferative states
     Post-splenectomy
HEREDITARY
     Hereditary eosinophilia
GASTROINTESTINAL DISEASES
     Chronic active hepatitis
     Ulcerative colitis
     Eosinophilic gastroenteritis
HYPEREOSINOPHILIC SYNDROMES
     Löfflers syndrome
     Eosinophilic leukemia
     Polyarteritis nodosa
OTHER
     Addison disease
     Ionizing radiation therapy
     Immune deficiency disorders (ie,
        Wiskott-Aldrich)
     Chronic peritoneal dialysis
     Dermatitis herpetiformis
     Cat scratch disease
     Allergic bronchopulmonary
        aspergillosis
     Sarcoidosis
     Thrombocytopenia - absent radius
        syndrome
     Familial reticuloendotheliosis
     Congenital heart disease

Modified from: *Hematology of Infancy and
Childhood*, Nathan DG, Oski FA (eds), 3rd Edition,
W.B. Saunders Company, Philadelphia, 1987, pp.814-815.

Pediatrics, Rudolph AM, Hoffman JIE (eds), 18th
Edition, Appleton & Lange, New York, 1987, p.1069.

CAUSES OF BASOPHILIA

HYPERSENSITIVITY REACTIONS
INFLAMMATORY
- Ulcerative colitis
- Juvenile rheumatoid arthritis

INFECTIONS
- Varicella
- Tuberculosis
- Influenza
- Chronic sinusitis

NEOPLASTIC
- Chronic myelocytic leukemia
- Chronic granulocytic leukemia
- Myelodysplastic syndromes
- Hodgkin disease

HEMATOLOGIC
- Iron deficiency anemia
- Sideroblastic anemia
- Some hemolytic anemias
- Polycythemia vera

DRUGS
- Estrogens
- Antithyroid medications

ENDOCRINE
- Hypothyroidism
- Ovulation
- Pregnancy

OTHER
- Chronic renal failure
- Ionizing radiation therapy
- Stress

Modified from: *Hematology of Infancy and Childhood*, Nathan DG, Oski FA (eds), 3rd Edition, W.B. Saunders Company, Philadelphia, 1987, pp.814-815.

CAUSES OF THROMBOCYTOPENIA IN THE NEONATE

DECREASED PRODUCTION OF PLATELETS
    Congenital megakaryocytic
     hypoplasia
     (TAR syndrome)
    Congenital infiltrative processes
     (congenital leukemia)
    Inherited thrombocytopenias
ABNORMAL DISTRIBUTION OF PLATELETS
    Splenomegaly
    Giant hemangioma
INCREASED PLATELET DESTRUCTION
    Immune-mediated destruction
    Isoimmunization
    Maternal antibody (ITP, SLE)
    Nonspecific destruction
    Sepsis
    Intravascular coagulation syndromes
     (DIC, NEC)
COMBINED INCREASED DESTRUCTION AND
  DECREASED PRODUCTION
    Intrauterine infections
    Inherited thrombocytopenias
     (Wiskott-Aldrich syndrome)

Modified from: Lightsey AL: *Pediatric Clinics of North America* 27(2):297, 1980.

DRUGS ASSOCIATED WITH THROMBOCYTOPENIA IN CHILDREN

ANTICONVULSANTS, SEDATIVES
    Diphenylhydantoin
    Carbamazepine
    Clonazepam
    Sodium valproate
    Primidone
ANTIBIOTICS
    Sulfisoxazole
    Trimethoprim sulfamethoxazole
    Para-aminosalicylate
    Rifampin
    Pentamidine
    Chloramphenicol

MISCELLANEOUS
        Cytotoxic agents
        Sulfonylureas
        Gold salts
        Penicillamine
        Quinidine

Modified from: Lightsey AL: *Pediatric Clinics of North America* 27(2):299, 1980.

CAUSES OF THROMBOCYTOSIS

MYELOPROLIFERATIVE SYNDROMES
        Essential thrombocythemia
        Polycythemia vera
        Chronic myelocytic leukemia
        Myeloid metaplasia
        5q-syndrome
        Idiopathic sideroblastic anemia
INFLAMMATORY STATES
        Acute infections
        Acute rheumatic fever
        Rheumatic arthritis
        Ankylosing spondylitis
        Ulcerative colitis
        Regional enteritis
        Celiac and sprue
        Tuberculosis
        Sarcoidosis
        Chronic hepatitis
        Chronic osteomyelitis
DRUG INDUCED
        Epinephrine
        Vinca alkaloid
        Therapy for iron deficiency or
          vitamin B_{12} deficiency
        Passively addicted neonates
IMMUNE DISORDERS
        Collagen vascular disorders
        Graft-versus-host disease
        Nephrotic syndrome
HEMATOLOGIC DISORDERS
        Iron deficiency
        Vitamin E deficiency
        Chronic hemolytic anemias and
          hemoglobinopathies
        "Rebound" following
          thrombocytopenia

NEOPLASMS
    Lymphomas
    Hodgkin disease
    Neuroblastoma
    Hepatoblastoma
    Other childhood solid tumors
    Carcinomas
SURGICAL OR FUNCTIONAL ASPLENIA
MISCELLANEOUS
    Following hemorrhage or
        gastrointestinal blood loss
    Following surgery
    Following exercise
    Caffey disease
    Kawasaki syndrome

Modified from: *Hematology of Infancy and Childhood*, Nathan DG, Oski FA (eds), 3rd Edition, W.B. Saunders Company, Philadelphia, 1987, p.1398.

CONDITIONS OR DISEASE ASSOCIATED WITH A HYPERCOAGULABLE STATE

ACUTE PERIPHERAL ARTERIAL INSUFFICIENCY
AGING
ANTITHROMBIN III DEFICIENCY
ARTERIOVENOUS SHUNTS
ATHEROSCLEROSIS
BEHCET DISEASE
BUERGER DISEASE
VASCULAR CATHETERS
CARDIOMYOPATHY, ATRIAL FIBRILLATION,
    MITRAL VALVE PROLAPSE
CHRONIC VALVULAR HEART DISEASE
CIGARETTE SMOKING
CROHN DISEASE
DEEP VEIN THROMBOSIS
DIABETES MELLITUS
DISSEMINATED INTRAVASCULAR COAGULATION
DYSFIBRINOGENEMIA
ESTROGEN THERAPY
FACTOR XII DEFICIENCY
GLOMERULAR DISEASE
HEMOLYTIC UREMIC SYNDROME
HEPARIN THERAPY
HOMOCYSTINURIA
HYPERCHOLESTEROLEMIA
HYPERBETALIPOPROTEINEMIA TYPE II
HYPOTHERMIA

KAWASAKI SYNDROME
LIVER DISEASE
LUPUS ANTICOAGULANT
MALIGNANCIES
MYELOPROLIFERATIVE SYNDROME
NEPHROTIC SYNDROME
NUTRITIONAL DEFICIENCIES (VITAMIN E
    DEFICIENCY, SELENIUM DEFICIENCY)
OXYGEN TOXICITY
PAROXYSMAL NOCTURNAL HEMOGLOBINURIA
PLACENTAL INSUFFICIENCY SYNDROME
PLASMINOGEN AND PLASMINOGEN ACTIVATOR
    ABNORMALITIES
POST MYOCARDIAL INFARCTION
POSTOPERATIVE STATES
POST STREPTOKINASE OR COUMARIN THERAPY
PROSTHETIC DEVICES IN THE CIRCULATION
PROSTACYCLIN OR PLASMA PROSTACYCLIN
    REGENERATING FACTOR DEFICIENCIES
PROTEIN C and S DEFICIENCIES
PREGNANCY
PREECLAMPSIA
RENAL ALLOGRAFT REJECTION
SICKLE CELL ANEMIA
STASIS
THROMBOTIC THROMBOCYTOPENIC PURPURA
TRANSIENT CEREBRAL ISCHEMIC ATTACKS
ULCERATIVE COLITIS
VASCULITIS
VENTRICULOJUGULAR SHUNTS

Modified from: *Hematology of Infancy and Childhood*
Nathan DG, Oski FA (eds), 3rd Edition, W.B. Saunders
Company, Philadelphia, 1987, p.1456.

DISEASES WITH ELEVATED SEDIMENTATION RATE

INFECTIONS
- Majority of bacterial infections
- Infectious hepatitis
- Cat scratch disease
- Post-perfusion syndrome
- Tuberculosis
- Secondary syphilis
- Leptospirosis
- Systemic fungal infections

HEMATOLOGIC AND NEOPLASTIC
- Severe anemia
- Leukemia
- Lymphoma
- Metastatic tumors
- Chronic granulomatous disease

GASTROINTESTINAL
- Ulcerative colitis
- Regional enteritis
- Acute pancreatitis
- Lupoid hepatitis
- Cholecystitis
- Peritonitis

COLLAGEN DISEASES
- Rheumatic fever
- Rheumatoid arthritis
- Lupus erythematosus
- Dermatomyositis
- Scleroderma
- Systemic vasculitis
- Henoch-Schönlein purpura
- Mediterranean fever

RENAL
- Acute glumerulonephritis
- Chronic glomerulonephritis with renal failure
- Nephrosis
- Pyelonephritis
- Hemolytic uremic syndrome

MISCELLANEOUS
- Hypothyroidism
- Thyroiditis
- Sarcoidosis
- Infantile cortical hyperostosis
- Surgery, burns

Modified from: Lascar AD: *Pediatric Clinics of North America* 19(4):1116, 1972.

DISORDERS THAT PRODUCE A LOW SEDIMENTATION RATE

ANOREXIA NERVOSA
HYPOFIBRINOGENEMIA
ABETALIPOPROTEINEMIA
SICKLE CELL ANEMIA
PYRUVATE KINASE DEFICIENCY
HEREDITARY SPHEROCYTOSIS
CONGESTIVE HEART FAILURE
NEPHROTIC SYNDROME
STEROID THERAPY
ASPIRIN ADMINISTRATION
SERUM SICKNESS

CHAPTER X

INFECTIOUS DISEASES

CAT AND DOG ASSOCIATED INFECTIONS

CATS

HUMAN ILLNESS	CAUSATIVE ORGANISM
Toxoplasmosis	Toxoplasma gondii
Dipylidiasis	Dipylidium caninum
Campylobacteriosis	Campylobacter jejuni
Tularemia	Francisella tularensis
Plague	Yersinia pestis
Cat scratch disease	Bacilli
Tinea or ringworm	Microsporum canis
Rabies	Rabies virus
Visceral larva migrans	Toxocara cati

DOGS

HUMAN ILLNESS	CAUSATIVE ORGANISM
Visceral larva migrans	Toxocara canis
Ocular larva migrans	Toxocara canis
Cutaneous larva migrans	Ancylostoma/caninum Ancylostoma brazilienze
Pulmonary dirofilariasis	Dirofilaria immitis
Echinococcosis	Echinococcus granulosus
Dipylidiasis	Dipylidium caninum
Brucellosis	Brucella canis
Leptospirosis	Leptospira canicola
Campylobacteriosis	Campylobacter jejuni
Salmonellosis	Salmonella (nontyphoidal)
Rocky Mountain Spotted Fever	Rickettsia rickettsii
Tularemia	Francisella tularensis
Tinea or ringworm	Microsporum canis
Rabies	Rabies virus

Modified from: Elliot DL, Tolle SW, Goldberg L, Miller JB: *N Engl J Med* 313:985-995, 1985.

PATHOGENS MOST COMMONLY ISOLATED FROM A DOG BITE

PASTEURELLA MULTOCIDA
STREPTOCOCCUS SPP
STAPHYLOCOCCUS AUREUS
PROPIONIBACTERIUM SPP
STAPHYLOCOCCUS EPIDERMIDIS
PEPTOCOCCUS SPP
BACTEROIDES SPP

Modified from: *Textbook of Pediatric Infectious Diseases*, Feigin RD, Cherry JD (eds), 2nd Edition, W.B. Saunders Company, Philadelphia, 1987, p.2363.

INFECTIOUS DISEASES OF HUMANS TRANSMITTED BY TICKS

DISEASE	AGENT
ENCEPHALITIS	ARBOVIRUS
BABESIOSIS	BABESIA MICROTI
LYME DISEASE	BORRELIA BURGDORFERI
RELAPSING FEVER	BORRELIA DUTTONII
	HERMISII
	TURICATAE
Q FEVER	COXIELLA BURNETTI
ERLICHIOSIS	ERLICHIA CANIS
	SENNETSU
TULAREMIA	FRANCISELLA TULARENSIS
COLORADO TICK FEVER	ORBIVIRUS
QUEENSLAND TICK TYPHUS	RICKETTSIA AUSTRALIS
FIEVRE BOUTONNEUSE	RICKETTSIA CONORII
ROCKY MOUNTAIN SPOTTED FEVER	RICKETTSIA RICKETTSII
ASIAN TICK TYPHUS	RICKETTSIA SIBERICUS

Modified from: *Textbook of Pediatric Infectious Diseases*, Feigin RD, Cherry JD (Eds), 2nd Edition, W.B. Saunders Company, Philadelphia, 1987, p.2134.

ANIMALS MOST COMMONLY TRANSMITTING RABIES

SKUNKS
RACCOONS
BATS
FARM ANIMALS
CATS
FOXES
DOGS

Modified from: *Textbook of Pediatric Infectious Diseases*, Feigin RD, Cherry JD (eds), 2nd Edition, W.B. Saunders Company, Philadelphia, 1987, p.1678.

CONDITIONS THAT PREDISPOSE TO CANDIDIASIS

INFANCY
PREGNANCY
HYPOVITAMINOSIS A
MALNUTRITION
IRON DEFICIENCY ANEMIA
BURNS
TRAUMA
DIABETES MELLITUS
ADDISON DISEASE
CUSHING SYNDROME
HYPOTHYROIDISM
HYPOPARATHYROIDISM
MALIGNANCY
INTRAVASCULAR CATHETERS
URINARY CATHETERS
IRRADIATION
SURGERY
ORGAN TRANSPLANTATION
CONGENITAL IMMUNE DEFICIENCY DISORDERS
ACQUIRED IMMUNODEFICIENCY SYNDROME

Modified from: *Textbook of Pediatric Infectious Diseases*, Feigin RD, Cherry JD (eds), 2nd Edition, W.B. Saunders Company, Philadelphia, 1987, p.1940.

MICROORGANISMS FOR WHICH PENICILLIN G IS THE DRUG OF CHOICE

STREPTOCOCCUS - GROUPS A, B, C, G
                          D (NON-ENTEROCOCCUS)
              - VIRIDANS GROUP
              - ANAEROBIC STRAINS
STREPTOCOCCUS PNEUMONIAE
STAPHYLOCOCCUS AUREUS AND EPIDERMIDIS
  (NON-BETA-LACTAMASE PRODUCING STRAINS)
NEISSERIA MENINGITIDIS
NEISSERIA GONORRHEA
TREPONEMA PALLIDUM
TREPONEMA PERTENUE
LEPTOSPIRA SPP
BACILLUS ANTHRACIS
CLOSTRIDIUM SPP
CORYNEBACTERIUM DIPHTHERIAE
BACTEROIDES SPP - OROPHARYNGEAL STRAINS
LEPTOTRICHIA BUCCALIS
PASTEURELLA MULTOCIDA
SPIRILLUM MINUS
STREPTOBACILLUS MONILIFORMIS
ACTINOMYCES ISRAELII

Modified from: *Textbook of Pediatric Infectious Diseases*, Feigin RD, Cherry JD (eds), 2nd Edition, W.B. Saunders Company, Philadelphia, 1987, p.2210.

JONES CRITERIA FOR DIAGNOSIS OF RHEUMATIC FEVER

MAJOR CRITERIA
     Carditis
     Arthritis
     Chorea
     Erythema marginatum
     Subcutaneous nodules
MINOR CRITERIA
     Previous rheumatic fever
     Arthralgia
     Fever
     Elevated ESR
     Elevated WBC count
     Prolongation of PR interval
     Presence of C-reactive protein

ETIOLOGIC AGENTS OF EXUDATIVE PHARYNGITIS

STREPTOCOCCUS PYOGENES (GROUP A)
CORYNEBACTERIUM DIPHTHERIAE
CORYNEBACTERIUM HEMOLYTICUM
FRANCISELLA TULARENSIS
ADENOVIRUSES
EPSTEIN-BARR VIRUS
CANDIDA SPP

Modified from: *Textbook of Pediatric Infectious Diseases*, Feigin RD, Cherry JD (eds), 2nd Edition, W.B. Saunders Company, Philadelphia, 1987, pp.182-183.

PATHOGENS ASSOCIATED WITH GASTROENTERITIS AND ARTHRITIS

SALMONELLA
SHIGELLA
YERSINIA
CAMPYLOBACTER
TUBERCULOSIS
ADENOVIRUS
ECHOVIRUS

Modified from: *Textbook of Pediatric Infectious Diseases*, Feigin RD, Cherry JD (eds), 2nd Edition, W.B. Saunders Company, Philadelphia, 1987, pp.182-183.

INFECTIOUS AGENTS ASSOCIATED WITH EXANTHEM AND MENINGITIS

HERPES SIMPLEX VIRUS 2
COXSACKIE VIRUSES A2, A9, B1, B4, B5
ECHO VIRUSES 4, 6, 9, 11, 14, 17, 25, 33
COLORADO TICK FEVER VIRUS
REOVIRUS 2
NEISSERIA MENINGITIDIS
LISTERIA MONOCYTOGENES
TOXOPLASMA GONDII

Modified from: *Textbook of Pediatric Infectious Diseases*, Feigin RD, Cherry JD (eds), 2nd Edition, W.B. Saunders Company, Philadelphia, 1987, p.810.

BACTERIAL CAUSES OF ACUTE GASTROENTERITIS

> SALMONELLA SPP
> SHIGELLA SPP
> CAMPYLOBACTER SPP
> E. COLI
> YERSINIA ENTEROCOLITICA
> CLOSTRIDIUM DIFFICILE
> AEROMONAS HYDROPHILA
> BACILLUS CEREUS
> STAPHYLOCOCCUS AUREUS
> VIBRIO CHOLERAE
> VIBRIO PARAHAEMOLYTICUS

Modified from: *Principles and Practice of Pediatrics*;
Oski FA, DeAngelis CD, Feigin RD, Warshaw JB (eds); JB
Lippincott Company, Philadelphia, 1990, p.1323.

CAUSES OF ATYPICAL LYMPHOCYTOSIS (GREATER THAN 20% OF WBC'S)

> INFECTIOUS MONONUCLEOSIS
> VIRAL HEPATITIS
> THE "POST-TRANSFUSION" SYNDROME
> PAS HYPERSENSITIVITY
> DILANTIN HYPERSENSITIVITY
> CYTOMEGALOVIRUS

Modified from: *The Best Of The Whole Pediatrician's
Catalog*, McMillan JA, Stockman JA, Nieburg PI, Oski FA
(eds), W.B. Saunders Company, Philadelphia, 1984, p.180.

PATHOGENS CAUSING PNEUMONIA AND RASH

> MYCOPLASMA PNEUMONIAE
> ATYPICAL MEASLES
> COXSACKIEVIRUS A9
> ECHOVIRUSES TYPES 6 AND 11
> REOVIRUS TYPE 3
> COCCIDIOIDOMYCOSIS
> ADENOVIRUS TYPE 7
> PSITTACOSIS
> INFECTIOUS MONONUCLEOSIS

Modified from: *The Whole Pediatrician*, McMillan JA,
Stockman JA III, Oski FA (eds), W.B. Saunders Company,
Philadelphia, 1979, p.160.

AGENTS PRODUCING PARINAUD OCULOGLANDULAR SYNDROME

EPSTEIN-BARR VIRUS
HERPES SIMPLEX VIRUS
CAT SCRATCH DISEASE
LEPTOTHRIX SPP
FRANCISELLA TULARENSIS
COCCIDIOIDES IMMITIS
YERSINIA SPP
TREPONEMA PALLIDUM
HEMOPHILUS DUCREYI
SPOROTRICHUM SCHENCKII
RHINOSPORIDUM SEEBERI
CHLAMYDIA TRACHOMATIS
ACTINOMYCES ISRAELII
MYCOBACTERIUM TUBERCULOSIS

Modified from: *Textbook of Pediatric Infectious Diseases*, Feigin RD, Cherry JD (eds), 2nd Edition, W.B. Saunders Company, Philadelphia, 1987, p.882.

CLINICAL INFECTIONS CAUSED BY ANAEROBES

PERITONITIS
WOUND INFECTION FOLLOWING ABDOMINAL
    SURGERY
BACTEREMIA ASSOCIATED WITH
    GASTROINTESTINAL DISEASE
SEPTICEMIA IN IMMUNOCOMPROMISED HOSTS
CERVICAL ADENITIS
OTITIS MEDIA
DENTAL ABSCESS
PERITONSILLAR ABSCESS
BRANCHIAL CLEFT CYST INFECTION
PARANASAL SINUSITIS
LUDWIG ANGINA
HUMAN AND ANIMAL BITES
SOFT TISSUE CELLULITIS
CHOLANGITIS
BRAIN ABSCESS

Modified from: *Textbook of Pediatric Infectious Diseases*, Feigin RD, Cherry JD (eds), 2nd Edition, W.B. Saunders Company, Philadelphia, 1987, p.1088.

CAUSES OF CSF EOSINOPHILIA

>PARASITIC INFECTION
NEUROSYPHILIS
COCCIDIOIDES IMMITIS MENINGITIS
POST RABIES VACCINATION
CANDIDA ALBICANS MENINGITIS
PNEUMOCOCCAL MENINGITIS
HODGKIN DISEASE
LYMPHOMA
FOREIGN PROTEIN IN THE CSF
RUBBER VENTRICULOATRIAL SHUNT
MULTIPLE SCLEROSIS-LIKE ILLNESS
LYMPHOCYTIC CHORIOMENINGITIS

Modified from: Chesney PJ, Katcher ML, Nelson DB, Horowitz SD: *J Pediatr* 94:750, 1979.

COMPLICATIONS OF INFECTIOUS MONONUCLEOSIS

>NEUROLOGIC
>>Guillain-Barré syndrome
Facial nerve palsy
Meningoencephalitis
Aseptic meningitis
Transverse myelitis
Seizures
Peripheral neuritis
Optic neuritis
Acute psychosis
Diplopia
Reye syndrome
Subacute sclerosing panencephalitis
>
>HEPATIC
>>Hepatitis
Multiple granulomas
>
>CARDIAC
>>Pericarditis
Myocarditis

HEMATOLOGIC
- Hemolytic anemia
- Thrombocytopenia
- Aplastic anemia
- Hemolytic-uremic syndrome
- Disseminated intravascular coagulation
- X-linked lymphoproliferative syndrome

SPLENIC RUPTURE
PULMONARY INFILTRATION
AIRWAY OBSTRUCTION
GLOMERULONEPHRITIS

Modified from: *The Whole Pediatrician's Catalog: A Compendium of Clues to Diagnosis and Management*, McMillan JA, Nieburg PI, Oski FA (eds), W.B. Saunders Company, Philadelphia, 1977, pp.178-179.

MANIFESTATIONS OF CONGENITAL RUBELLA

DEAFNESS
CONGENITAL HEART DISEASE
PSYCHOMOTOR RETARDATION
RETINOPATHY
CATARACTS
NEONATAL PURPURA
GLAUCOMA

Modified from: *Textbook of Pediatric Infectious Diseases*, Feigin RD, Cherry JD (eds), 2nd Edition, W.B. Saunders Company, Philadelphia, 1987, p.984.

MANIFESTATIONS OF CONGENITAL TOXOPLASMOSIS

        ABNORMAL CSF
        CHORIORETINITIS
        STRABISMUS
        INTRACRANIAL CALCIFICATIONS
        PREMATURITY
        JAUNDICE
        ABNORMAL EEG
        INTRAUTERINE GROWTH RETARDATION
        HYPOTONIA
        PSYCHOMOTOR RETARDATION
        MICROCEPHALY
        ABNORMAL CBC
        HEPATOSPLENOMEGALY
        CONVULSIONS
        MICROPHTHALMIA
        HYDROCEPHALY
        PURPURA

Modified from: *Textbook of Pediatric Infectious Diseases*, Feigin RD, Cherry JD (eds), 2nd Edition, W.B. Saunders Company, Philadelphia, 1987, p.2071.

MANIFESTATIONS OF EARLY CONGENITAL SYPHILIS

        HEPATOMEGALY
        SKELETAL ABNORMALITIES
        BIRTH WEIGHT < 2500 G
        SKIN LESIONS
        HYPERBILIRUBINEMIA
        PNEUMONIA
        SPLENOMEGALY
        SEVERE ANEMIA, HYDROPS
        SNUFFLES
        PAINFUL LIMBS
        PANCREATITIS
        CSF ABNORMALITIES
        NEPHRITIS/NEPHROSIS
        FAILURE TO THRIVE

Modified from: *Textbook of Pediatric Infectious Diseases*, Feigin RD, Cherry JD (eds), 2nd Edition, W.B. Saunders Company, Philadelphia, 1987, p.613.

STIGMATA OF LATE CONGENITAL SYPHILIS

> FRONTAL BOSS OF PARROTT
> SHORT MAXILLA
> HIGH PALATAL ARCH
> SADDLE NOSE
> MULBERRY MOLARS
> HUTCHINSON TEETH
> HIGOUMENAKIS SIGN
> RELATIVE PROTUBERANCE OF MANDIBLE
> RHAGADES
> SABER SHIN

Modified from: *Textbook of Pediatric Infectious Diseases*, Feigin RD, Cherry JD (eds), 2nd Edition, W.B. Saunders Company, Philadelphia, 1987, p.613.

MANIFESTATIONS OF CONGENITAL CYTOMEGALOVIRUS INFECTION

> LOW BIRTH WEIGHT
> HEPATOMEGALY
> SPLENOMEGALY
> JAUNDICE
> PETECHIAE, PURPURA
> MICROCEPHALY
> PNEUMONIA
> RETINOPATHY
> CEREBRAL CALCIFICATIONS

Modified from: *Textbook of Pediatric Infectious Diseases*, Feigin RD, Cherry JD (eds), 2nd Edition, W.B. Saunders Company, Philadelphia, 1987, p.974.

MANIFESTATIONS OF CONGENITAL VARICELLA

> OCULAR ABNORMALITIES
> LIMB HYPOPLASIA
> CUTANEOUS SCARS
> PREMATURITY
> CORTICAL ATROPHY
> BULBAR PALSY

Modified from: *Textbook of Pediatric Infectious Diseases*, Feigin RD, Cherry JD (eds), 2nd Edition, W.B. Saunders Company, Philadelphia, 1987, p.996.

MANIFESTATIONS OF CONGENITAL HERPES SIMPLEX

VESICULAR RASH
LOW BIRTH WEIGHT
CHORIORETINITIS
DIFFUSE BRAIN DAMAGE
MICROCEPHALY
INTRACRANIAL CALCIFICATIONS
MICROPHTHALMIA
CATARACTS
RETINAL DYSPLASIA

Modified from: *Textbook of Pediatric Infectious Diseases*, Feigin RD, Cherry JD (eds), 2nd Edition, W.B. Saunders Company, Philadelphia, 1987, p.990.

INDIVIDUALS FOR WHOM PRE-EXPOSURE PROPHYLAXIS WITH HEPATITIS B VIRUS VACCINE IS RECOMMENDED

HEALTH CARE WORKERS
STAFF AT INSTITUTIONS FOR MENTALLY RETARDED
HEMODIALYSIS PATIENTS
RECIPIENT OF BLOOD PRODUCTS
HOMOSEXUALLY ACTIVE MALES
ILLICIT DRUG USERS
HOUSEHOLD SEXUAL CONTACTS OF HBV CARRIERS
LONG-TERM INMATES OF CORRECTIONAL FACILITIES
IMMIGRANTS FROM AREAS WHERE HBV IS HIGHLY ENDEMIC

Modified from: *Textbook of Pediatric Infectious Diseases*, Feigin RD, Cherry JD (eds), 2nd Edition, W.B. Saunders Company, Philadelphia, 1987, p.736.

VACCINES AND TOXOIDS COMMERCIALLY AVAILABLE IN THE U.S.

    BCG
    CHOLERA
    DIPHTHERIA TOXOID
    DIPHTHERIA AND TETANUS TOXOID (DT FOR
      PEDIATRIC USE)
    DTP
    HEMOPHILUS b POLYSACCHARIDE
    HEMOPHILUS b POLYSACCHARIDE, DIPHTHERIA
      TOXOID CONJUGATE
    HEPATITIS B VACCINES
            Plasma Derived
            Recombinant
    INFLUENZA VIRUS VACCINE
    MEASLES VIRUS VACCINE
    MEASLES AND RUBELLA VIRUS VACCINE
    MEASLES, MUMPS, AND RUBELLA VIRUS
      VACCINE
    MENINGOCOCCAL POLYSACCHARIDE
    MUMPS VIRUS VACCINE
    PLAGUE VACCINE
    POLIOVIRUS VACCINE (INACTIVATED)
    POLIOVIRUS VACCINE (LIVE, ORAL)
    PNEUMOCOCCAL POLYSACCHARIDE
    RABIES VACCINE
    RUBELLA VIRUS VACCINE
    RUBELLA AND MUMPS VIRUS
    STAPHYLOCOCCAL BACTERIAL ANTIGEN
    TETANUS AND DIPHTHERIA TOXOIDS (Td, FOR
      ADULT USE)
    TETANUS TOXOID
    TYPHOID VACCINE
    YELLOW FEVER VACCINE

Modified from: *Principles and Practice of Pediatrics*, Oski FA, DeAngelis CD, Feigin RD, Warshaw JB (eds), J.B. Lippincott Company, Philadelphia, 1990, p.554.

CONTRAINDICATIONS TO PERTUSSIS IMMUNIZATION

ABSOLUTE
    Previous occurrences of adverse side
        effects:
            Persistent screaming > 3 hours
            High fever (>40.5C) in first 2
                days
            Unusual, high-pitched cry in first
                2 days
            Convulsion in first 3 days
            Collapse or shock in first 2 days
            Encephalopathy in first 7 days
    Prior allergic reaction to the vaccine
RELATIVE
    History of culture-proven pertussis
    Intercurrent febrile illness
    Children with evolving neurologic
        disorders
    Children with seizure disorder
    Children with progressive developmental
        delay

Modified from: *Red Book*, Report of the Committee on
Infectious Diseases, 21st Edition, American Academy of
Pediatrics, Evanston, 1988, pp.321-324.

CHILDREN WHO SHOULD RECEIVE THE
PNEUMOCOCCAL VACCINE

CHILDREN $\geq$ 2 YEARS WITH:
    SICKLE CELL ANEMIA
    ASPLENIA
    NEPHROTIC SYNDROME
    HODGKIN DISEASE UNDERGOING
        THERAPY
    HIV INFECTION

Modified from: *Red Book*, Report of the Committee on
Infectious Diseases, 21st Edition, American Academy of
Pediatrics, Evanston, 1988, p.331.

IMMUNIZATION GUIDELINES FOR CHILDREN WITH HIV INFECTION

CHILDREN WITH SYMPTOMATIC INFECTION
      Avoid live viral (MMR, OPV) and live bacterial (BCG) vaccines
      Administer IPV instead of OPV
      Administer DTP and HIB vaccine on usual schedule
      Administer inactivated influenza vaccine annually to those > 6 months
      Administer pneumococcal vaccine once to those $\geq$ 24 months
      Administer immune globulin (IG) or varicella-zoster immune globulin (VZIG) following exposure to measles or varicella, respectively

CHILDREN WITH ASYMPTOMATIC INFECTION
      Administer MMR on usual schedule
      Administer IPV instead of OPV
      Administer DTP and HIB on usual schedule

CHILDREN RESIDING IN HOUSEHOLD OF PATIENT WITH HIV INFECTION
      Administer IPV instead of OPV

Modified from: *MMWR*; 35:595-606, 1986.

CLINICAL MANIFESTATIONS IN SYMPTOMATIC PEDIATRIC HIV INFECTION

LYMPHADENOPATHY
HEPATOMEGALY
SPLENOMEGALY
FAILURE TO THRIVE
SERIOUS BACTERIAL INFECTIONS
THRUSH; CANDIDAL DIAPER RASH
RECURRENT OTITIS MEDIA
NEUROLOGIC ABNORMALITIES
OPPORTUNISTIC INFECTIONS

LYMPHOCYTIC INTERSTITIAL PNEUMONITIS
DIARRHEA
MICROCEPHALY
CLUBBING OF NAILS
SALIVARY GLAND ENLARGEMENT
LYMPHOMA

Modified from: Falloon J, Eddy J, Wiener L, Pizzo PA: *J Pediatr* 114:10, 1989.

ORGANISMS TRANSMITTED THROUGH BREAST MILK

CYTOMEGALOVIRUS
HEPATITIS B VIRUS
HUMAN IMMUNODEFICIENCY VIRUS
TRYPANISOMIASIS

Modified from: *Redbook*, Report of the Committee on Infectious Diseases, 21st Edition, American Academy of Pediatrics, Evanston, 1988.

Dworsky M, et al: *Pediatrics* 72:295-299, 1983.

THE SIX "CLASSIC" CHILDHOOD EXANTHEMS

FIRST DISEASE	RUBEOLA OR MEASLES
SECOND DISEASE	SCARLET FEVER
THIRD DISEASE	RUBELLA OR GERMAN MEASLES
FOURTH DISEASE	FILATOW-DUKES DISEASE*
FIFTH DISEASE	ERYTHEMA INFECTIOSUM (PARVO B_{19})
SIXTH DISEASE	EXANTHEM SUBITUM OR ROSEOLA INFANTUM

*   Not a separate disease but a variant of
    scarlet fever or of toxin producing
    staphylococci.

Modified from: Feder HM, Anderson I; *Arch Int Med* 149:2176, 1989.

COUNTRIES WITH REPORTED CHLOROQUINE-RESISTANT MALARIA

AFRICA
  ANGOLA
  BENIN
  BURUNDI
  CAMEROON
  CENTRAL AFRICAN
    REPUBLIC
  COMOROS
  CONGO
  GABON
  KENYA
  MADAGASCAR
  MALAWI
  MOZAMBIQUE
  NAMIBIA
  NIGERIA
  RWANDA
  SOUTH AFRICA
  SUDAN
  SWAZILAND
  TANZANIA
  UGANDA
  ZAIRE
  ZAMBIA
  ZIMBABWE
OCEANIA
  PAPUA NEW GUINEA
  SOLOMON ISLANDS
  VANUATU

SOUTH/CENTRAL AMERICA
  BOLIVIA
  BRAZIL
  COLOMBIA
  EQUADOR
  FRENCH GUIANA
  GUYANA
  PANAMA
  PERU
  SURINAM
  VENEZUELA

ASIA
  BANGLADESH
  BURMA
  CHINA
  INDIA
  INDONESIA
  KAMPUCHEA
  LAOS
  MALAYSIA
  PAKISTAN
  PHILIPPINES
  SRI LANKA
  THAILAND
  VIET NAM

Modified from: Report of the Committee on Infectious
Diseases, American Academy of Pediatrics; 1989:275.

CHAPTER XI

NEONATOLOGY

EVENTS ASSOCIATED WITH SPONTANEOUS PREMATURE BIRTH

MATERNAL FACTORS
History of previous premature birth
Malnutrition
Uterine abnormalities
Uterine stretch (hydramnios)
Age less than 16 years or over 35 years
Cyanotic heart disease and other chronic diseases
Short interval between births
Infection
Trauma
Hypertension
Diethylstilbestrol exposure

FETAL FACTORS
Malformations
Multiple births
Premature rupture of membranes

ENVIRONMENTAL EFFECTS
Lower socioeconomic class

HABITS
Smoking
Fatigue/activity
Cocaine use

Modified from: *Schaffer's Diseases of the Newborn*,
Avery ME, Taeusch HW (eds), 5th Edition, W.B. Saunders
Company, Philadelphia, 1984, p.83.

FETAL ABNORMALITIES DIAGNOSED BY ULTRASONOGRAPHY

HYDROCEPHALY
HYDRANENCEPHALY
ANENCEPHALY
MYELOMENINGOCELE
CONJOINED TWINS
FETAL HEART STRUCTURAL ABNORMALITIES
HEART RATE ABNORMALITIES
Tachycardia
Bradycardia
UPPER GASTROINTESTINAL OBSTRUCTION
FETAL DEATH
ASCITES/HYDROPS
OMPHALOCELE

DIAPHRAGMATIC HERNIA
MULTICYSTIC KIDNEYS
URINARY OBSTRUCTION
RENAL AGENESIS
SKELETAL DYSPLASIAS
PLACENTA PREVIA
ABRUPTIO PLACENTAE

Modified from: *Schaffer's Diseases of the Newborn*,
Avery ME, Taeusch HW (eds), 5th Edition, W.B. Saunders
Company, Philadelphia, 1984, p.83.

FETAL ANOMALIES SEEN WITH ELEVATED AMNIOTIC FLUID ALPHA-FETOPROTEIN

PROBABLE
Anencephaly
Open spina bifida
Fetal demise
Exophthalmos
Congenital nephrosis
Fetal teratoma
Seckel syndrome
Extrophy of cloaca
POSSIBLE
Esophageal atresia
Duodenal atresia
Turner syndrome
Fetus papyraceous
Gastroschisis
Congenital skin defects
Conjoined twins
Hemangioma of umbilical cord

Modified from: *Neonatology Pathophysiology and Management
of the Newborn*, Avery GB (ed), J.B. Lippincott Company,
Philadelphia, 1987, p.142.

SELECTED MATERNAL CONDITIONS ASSOCIATED WITH ELEVATED ALPHA-FETOPROTEIN

HEPATOCARCINOMA AND OTHER TUMORS
LIVER CELL REGENERATION
TYROSINEMIA
ATAXIA-TELANGIECTASIA

Modified from: *Schaffer's Diseases of the Newborn*,
Avery ME, Taeusch HW (eds), 5th Edition, W.B. Saunders
Company, Philadelphia, 1984, p.29.

SINGLE UMBILICAL ARTERY

FREQUENT IN
    Extrophy of bladder
    Monozygotic twinning
    Sirenomelia sequence
    Vater association
OCCASIONAL IN
    Fetal hydantoin effects
    Jarcho-Levis syndrome
    Meckel-Gruber syndrome
    Multiple lentigines syndrome
    Trisomy 13 syndrome
    Trisomy 18 syndrome
    Zellweger syndrome

Modified from: Smith's Recognizable Patterns of Human
Malformation, Jones KL (ed), 4th Edition, W.B.
Saunders Company, Philadelphia, 1988, p.755.

CLINICAL CONDITIONS ASSOCIATED WITH HYDRAMNIOS

AGNATHIA
    Microstomia synotia syndrome
AMINOPTERIN SYNDROME
ANENCEPHALY AND OTHER CNS DEFECTS
ARTHROGRYPOSIS
BECKWITH-WIEDEMANN SYNDROME
CONGENITAL CHYLOTHORAX
CONJOINED TWINS
DIAPHRAGMATIC HERNIA

FETAL DEATH
FETAL HYDROPS
GASTROSCHISIS
HEMANGIOMA
MATERNAL DIABETES
TERATOMAS
TRISOMIES
TUMORS
UMBILICAL CORD COMPRESSION
UPPER GASTROINTESTINAL OBSTRUCTION
WERDNIG-HOFFMANN DISEASE

Modified from: *Schaffer's Diseases of the Newborn*,
Avery ME, Taeusch HW (eds), 5th Edition, W.B. Saunders
Company, Philadelphia, 1984, p.19.

SOME FINDINGS ASSOCIATED WITH INTRAUTERINE GROWTH RETARDATION

MATERNAL FACTORS
 Infections
  Rubella
  Cytomegalovirus
  Toxoplasmosis
  Syphilis
 Toxemia
 Chronic hypertension
 Cyanotic heart disease
 Short stature (height less than
  150 cm)
 Primiparity
 Severe malnutrition
 Cigarette smoking
 Narcotic usage
 Low maternal age
 Previous baby 2.5 kg or less
ENVIRONMENTAL FACTORS
 Residence at high altitude
 Radiation
 Exposure to teratogens

PLACENTAL FACTORS
    Infarcts
    Thrombosis of fetal vessels
    Single umbilical artery
    Premature partial separation
    Twin-twin transfusion
FETAL FACTORS
    Twins (multiple pregnancy)
    Chromosomal abnormalities
    Other congenital malformations
    Inborn errors of metabolism
    Insulin deficiency

Modified from: *Schaffer's Diseases of the Newborn*, Avery ME, Taeusch HW (eds), 5th Edition, W.B. Saunders Company, Philadelphia, 1984, p.95.

TYPES OF HEMORRHAGE IN THE FETUS AND NEWBORN

OCCULT HEMORRHAGE PRIOR TO BIRTH
    Fetomaternal
        Traumatic amniocentesis
        Spontaneous
        Following external cephalic
            version
    Twin-twin
OBSTETRIC ACCIDENTS, MALFORMATIONS OF
THE PLACENTA AND CORD
    Rupture of normal umbilical cord
        Precipitous delivery
        Entanglement
    Hematoma of the cord or placenta
    Rupture of an abnormal umbilical
      cord
        Varices
        Aneurysm
    Rupture of anomalous vessels
        Aberrant vessel
        Velamentous insertion
        Communicating vessels in
            multilobed placenta
    Incision of placenta during
      cesarean section
    Placenta previa
    Abruptio placentae

INTERNAL HEMORRHAGE
    Intracranial
    Giant cephalohematoma
    Caput succedaneum
    Retroperitoneal
    Ruptured liver
    Ruptured spleen

Modified from: *Neonatology Pathophysiology and Management of the Newborn*, Avery GB (ed), 3rd Edition, J.B. Lippincott Company, Philadelphia, 1987, p.645.

CAUSES OF HYDROPS FETALIS

INFECTIONS
    Toxoplasmosis
    Cytomegalic inclusion virus
    Leptospirosis
    Chagas disease
    Syphilis
    Parvovirus
    Congenital hepatitis
CHRONIC ANEMIA
    Blood group incompatibility
    Alpha thalassemia
    G6PD deficiency
    Gaucher disease
    Parabiotic syndrome
    Chronic fetomaternal transfusion
CARDIAC DISEASE OR FAILURE
    Severe congenital heart disease
    Fetal arrhythmias
    Large A-V malformation
    Premature closure of foramen ovale
    Cardiopulmonary hypoplasia with
        bilateral hydrothorax
    Premature closure of ductus arteriosus
        with hypoplasia of lungs
    Calcific myocarditis (Coxsackie virus)
    Cardiac neoplasm
    Twin pregnancy with "parasitic fetus"
    Myocarditis

RENAL DISEASE
    Congenital nephrosis
    Renal vein thrombosis
MALFORMATIONS AND CONGENITAL TUMORS
    Pulmonary hypoplasia
    Hemangioendothelioma
    Chorioangioma of the placenta
    Aneurysm of the umbilical artery
    Angiomyxoma of the umbilical cord
    Congenital neuroblastoma
    Cystic hygroma
    Cervical teratoma
    Pulmonary lymphangiectasia
    Cystic adenomatoid malformation of
        the lung
    Down syndrome
    Turner syndrome
    Sacrococcygeal teratoma
MATERNAL DISORDERS
    Diabetes mellitus
    Toxemia of pregnancy
    Polyhydramnios
IDIOPATHIC

Modified from: *Schaffer's Diseases of the Newborn*,
Avery ME, Taeusch HW (eds), 5th Edition, W.B. Saunders
Company, Philadelphia, 1984, p.636.

FACTORS AFFECTING INSENSIBLE WATER LOSS IN NEWBORN INFANTS

LEVEL OF MATURITY
> Inversely proportional to birth weight and gestational age

RESPIRATORY DISTRESS (HYPERPNEIC)
> IWL increases with rising minute ventilation when breathing dry air

ENVIRONMENTAL TEMPERATURE ABOVE NEUTRAL THERMAL ZONE
> Increases in proportion to increment in temperature

ELEVATED BODY TEMPERATURE
> Increased by up to 300%

SKIN BREAKDOWN OR INJURY
> Increased by uncertain magnitude

CONGENITAL SKIN DEFECTS (i.e. GASTROSCHISIS)
> Increased by uncertain magnitude

RADIANT WARMER
> Increased by about 50%

PHOTOTHERAPY
> Increased by about 50%

MOTOR ACTIVITY AND CRYING
> Increased by up to 70%

HIGH AMBIENT OR INSPIRED HUMIDITY
> Reduced by 30% when ambient vapor pressure is increased by 200%

PLASTIC HEAT SHIELD
> Reduced by 10% to 30%

Modified from: *Neonatology Pathophysiology and Management of the Newborn*, Avery GB (ed), 3rd Edition, J.B. Lippincott Company, Philadelphia, 1987, p.777.

COMPLICATIONS ASSOCIATED WITH INTRALIPID

ALLERGIC REACTION
HEPATOMEGALY
ADVERSE REACTION
> Hyperthermia
> Shock

EOSINOPHILIA
BLOOD HYPERCOAGULABILITY
REDUCTION OF PLATELET ADHESIVENESS
INTERFERENCE WITH BILIRUBIN MEASUREMENT

Modified from: *Care of the High Risk Neonate*, Klaus MH, Fanaroff AA (eds), 3rd Edition, W.B. Saunders Company, Philadelphia, 1986, p.133.

CAUSES OF INDIRECT HYPERBILIRUBINEMIA IN NEONATE

FETAL-MATERNAL BLOOD GROUP
  INCOMPATIBILITY
      Rh
      ABO
      Others
HEREDITARY SPHEROCYTOSIS
NONSPHEROCYTIC HEMOLYTIC ANEMIAS
      G-6-PD deficiency and drugs
      Pyruvate kinase deficiency
      Other red cell enzyme deficiencies
      Alpha-Thalassemia
      Beta-gamma thalassemia
      Vitamin K_3 induced hemolysis
EXTRAVASATION OF BLOOD
      Petechiae
      Hematoma
      Pulmonary
      Cerebral
      Occult hemorrhage
POLYCYTHEMIA
      Maternal-fetal transfusion
      Fetal-fetal transfusion
      Delayed clamping of cord
SWALLOWED BLOOD
INFANTS OF DIABETIC MOTHERS
INCREASED ENTEROHEPATIC CIRCULATION OF
  BILIRUBIN
      Pyloric stenosis
      Small bowel obstruction
      Large bowel obstruction
      Ileus
INBORN ERRORS OF METABOLISM
      Familial nonhemolytic jaundice
          Type I (Crigler-Najjar)
          Type II
      Gilbert syndrome
      Galactosemia
      Tyrosinosis
      Hypermethionemia
DRUGS AND HORMONES
      Hypothyroidism
      Hypopituitarism
      Anencephaly
      Lucey-Driscoll syndrome
      Breast milk jaundice

PREMATURITY
PHYSIOLOGIC JAUNDICE

Modified from: Maisels MJ: *Pediatrics in Review*
3:305-319, 1982.

CAUSES OF PROLONGED INDIRECT HYPERBILIRUBINEMIA

BREAST MILK JAUNDICE
HEMOLYTIC DISEASE
HYPOTHYROIDISM
PYLORIC STENOSIS
CRIGLER-NAJJAR SYNDROME
EXTRAVASCULAR BLOOD

Modified from: *Neonatology Pathophysiology and
Management of the Newborn*, Avery GB (ed), 3rd
Edition, J.B. Lippincott Company, Philadelphia,
1987, p.566.

DISORDERS OF THE NEWBORN INFANT ASSOCIATED WITH DIRECT HYPERBILIRUBINEMIA

OBSTRUCTION TO BILIARY FLOW
        Extrahepatic biliary atresia
        Paucity of intrahepatic ductules
          (intrahepatic biliary atresia)
        Choledochal cyst (bile duct stenosis)
        Bile-plug syndrome (inspissated bile
          syndrome)
        Cystic fibrosis
        Choledocholithiasis
        Tumors
        Hepatic hemangioendotheliomas
        Lymphadenopathy
HEPATIC CELL INJURY
        Infection
                Bacterial
                        Syphilis
                        Listeriosis
                        Tuberculosis

Viral
    Rubella
    Cytomegalovirus
    Herpes
    Coxsackie B
    (?) Hepatitis B
    (?) Hepatitis A
Parasitic
    Toxoplasmosis
Idiopathic
    Neonatal hepatitis (giant cell hepatitis)
TOXIC
    Bacterial sepsis (E. coli, Proteus, Pneumococcus)
    Intravenous alimentation
    Drugs
METABOLIC ERRORS
    Galactosemia
    Fructosemia
    Tyrosinemia
    Alpha-1-Antitrypsin deficiency
    Cystic fibrosis
    Infantile Gaucher disease
    Glycogenosis type IV
    Wolman disease
    Idiopathic neonatal hemochromatosis
    Niemann-Pick disease
    Cerebro-hepato-renal syndrome (Zellweger disease)
    Byler disease
    Trihydroxycoprostanic acidemia
    Indian childhood cirrhosis (?)
    Rotor syndrome
    Dubin-Johnson syndrome
CHRONIC BILIRUBIN OVERLOAD
    Erythroblastosis fetalis
    Glucose-6-phosphate dehydrogenase deficiency and other erythrocyte enzyme deficiencies
    Spherocytosis, elliptocytosis, pyknocytosis
    Congenital erythropoietic porphyria

Modified from: *Schaffer's Diseases of the Newborn*, Avery ME, Taeusch HW (eds), 5th Edition, W.B. Saunders Company, Philadelphia, 1984, p.644.

CLINICAL AND LABORATORY FEATURES OF ISOIMMUNE HEMOLYSIS DUE TO Rh DISEASE AND ABO INCOMPATIBILITY

	Rh	ABO
CLINICAL FEATURES		
Frequency	Unusual	Common
Pallor	Marked	Minimal
Jaundice	Marked	Minimal to moderate
Hydrops	Common	Rare
Hepatosplenomegaly	Marked	Minimal
LABORATORY FEATURES		
Blood type		
Mother	Rh (-)	0 (Most common)
Infant	Rh (+)	A or B
Anemia	Marked	Minimal
Direct Coomb's test	Positive	Frequently negative
Indirect Coomb's test	Positive	Usually positive
Hyperbilirubinemia	Marked	Variable
RBC morphology	Nucleated RBC's	Spherocytes

Modified from: *Schaffer's Diseases of the Newborn*, Avery ME, Taeusch HW (eds), 5th Edition, W.B. Saunders Company, Philadelphia, 1984, p.591.

HEMOLYTIC ANEMIA DURING THE NEWBORN PERIOD

```
IMMUNE
    Isoimmune
        Rh incompatibility
        ABO incompatibility
    Maternal immune disease
        Autoimmune hemolytic anemia
        Systemic lupus erythematosus
    Drug induced
        Penicillin
ACQUIRED RBC DISORDERS
    Membrane defects
        Hereditary spherocytosis
        Hereditary elliptocytosis
    Enzyme abnormalities
        G-6-PD
        Pyruvate kinase
```

> Hemoglobinopathies
>> Alpha thalassemia
>> Gamma/beta thalassemia

Modified from: *Schaffer's Diseases of the Newborn*,
Avery ME, Taeusch HW (eds), 5th Edition, W.B. Saunders
Company, Philadelphia, 1984, p.589.

COMPLICATIONS OF EXCHANGE TRANSFUSIONS

VASCULAR
  Embolization with air or thrombi
  Thrombosis
CARDIAC
  Arrhythmias
  Volume overload
  Arrest
ELECTROLYTE
  Hyperkalemia
  Hypernatremia
  Hypocalcemia
  Acidosis
COAGULATION
  Overheparinization
  Thrombocytopenia
INFECTIOUS
  Bacteremia
  Hepatitis
  Cytomegalovirus
OTHER
  Mechanical injury to donor cells
  Necrotizing enterocolitis
  Hypothermia
  Hypoglycemia

Modified from: *Care of the High Risk
Neonate*, Klaus MH, Fanaroff AA (eds), 3rd
Edition, W.B. Saunders Company, Philadelphia,
1986, p.253.

COMPLICATIONS OF PHOTOTHERAPY

    TANNING
    BRONZE BABY SYNDROME
    DIARRHEA
    LACTOSE INTOLERANCE
    HEMOLYSIS
    SKIN BURNS
    DEHYDRATION
    SKIN RASHES

Modified from: *Care of the High Risk Neonate*, Klaus MH, Fanaroff AA (eds), 3rd Edition, W.B. Saunders Company, Philadelphia, 1986, p.255.

CAUSES OF CONGESTIVE HEART FAILURE IN THE FIRST WEEK OF LIFE

    TRANSIENT MYOCARDIAL ISCHEMIA
    DYSRHYTHMIAS
    ARTERIOVENOUS FISTULA
    COARCTATION OF THE AORTA
    AORTIC STENOSIS
    HYPOPLASTIC LEFT HEART SYNDROME
    MYOCARDITIS

Modified from: *Schaffer's Diseases of the Newborn*, Avery ME, Taeusch HW (eds), 5th Edition, W.B. Saunders Company, Philadelphia, 1984, p.287.

CAUSES OF CONGESTIVE HEART FAILURE DURING THE SECOND THROUGH FOURTH WEEKS OF LIFE

    ACYANOTIC
        Coarctation of the aorta
        Aortic stenosis
        Myocarditis
        Endocardial fibroelastosis
        Patent ductus arteriosus
        Aortopulmonary window
        Arteriovenus fistula
        Ventricular septal defect (VSD)
        Endocardial cushion defect

CYANOTIC
>   Hypoplastic left heart syndrome
>   Total anomalous pulmonary venous
>   return
>   Truncus arteriosus
>   Transposition and a VSD
>   Tricuspid atresia and a VSD
>   Single ventricle

Modified from: *Schaffer's Diseases of the Newborn*,
Avery ME, Taeusch HW (eds), 5th Edition, W.B. Saunders
Company, Philadelphia, 1984, p.287.

CAUSES OF APNEA IN AN INFANT

COMMON CAUSES
>   Breath-holding spells
>   Gastroesophageal reflux
>   Idiopathic
>   Prematurity
>   Seizure

OCCASIONAL CAUSES
>   BPD "spells"
>   CNS trauma/bleed
>   Congenital airway abnormality
>   Congenital heart disease
>   Hypoglycemia
>   Hypoxia
>   Hypothermia
>   Infection
>>   Croup
>>   Meningitis
>>   Pneumonia
>>   Sepsis
>>   RSV
>   Laryngospasm
>   Laryngo-tracheo-bronchomalacia
>   Obstructive sleep apnea
>   SIDS
>   Toxins/drugs
>>   Sedatives, magnesium
>   Vascular abnormality causing airway
>   compression

RARE CAUSES
- Anemia
- Arrhythmia
- CNS structural lesions
- Central respiratory mechanism immaturity
- Hypocalcemia
- Increased ICP
- Intraventricular hemorrhage
- Inborn errors of metabolism

Modified from: *Principles and Practice of Pediatrics*, Oski FA, DeAngelis CD, Feigin RD, Warshaw JB (eds), J.B. Lippincott Company, Philadelphia, 1990, p.2026.

Ambulatory Pediatric Care, Dershewitz RA (ed), J.B. Lippincott Company, Philadelphia, 1988, p.844.

INDICATIONS FOR HOME APNEA MONITORING

INFANTS WITH ONE OR MORE SEVERE APPARENT
LIFE-THREATENING EPISODES REQUIRING
VIGOROUS RESUSCITATION OR STIMULATION
AND FOR WHOM NO TREATABLE CAUSE CAN
BE IDENTIFIED
INFANTS WITH TRACHEOSTOMY UNDER ONE YEAR OLD
INFANTS WITH BPD ON SUPPLEMENTAL OXYGEN
INFANTS WITH POTENTIALLY TREATABLE CAUSES OF
ALTE IN ORDER TO ASSESS RESPONSE TO
THERAPY OR UNTIL EFFECTIVENESS OF
THERAPY IS ESTABLISHED
PREMATURE INFANTS DISCHARGED ON XANTHINE
THERAPY FOR PERSISTENT APNEA
INFANTS OF COCAINE ABUSING MOTHERS
SIBLINGS OF 2 OR MORE SIDS VICTIMS

Modified from: Brooks JG: *Pediatrician* 15:212-216, 1988.

Principles and Practice of Pediatrics, Oski FA, DeAngelis CD, Feigin RD, Warshaw JB (eds), J.B. Lippincott Company, Philadelphia, 1990, p.979.

SEIZURES OCCURRING IN THE FIRST 10 DAYS OF LIFE

BIRTH TO DAY THREE
Perinatal complications
Hypoglycemia
Hypocalcemia
Developmental anomalies
DAY FOUR TO DAY TEN
Hypocalcemia
Infection
Developmental anomalies

Modified from: *Neonatology Pathophysiology and Management of the Newborn*, Avery GB (ed), 3rd Edition, J.B. Lippincott Company, Philadelphia, 1987, p.1087.

COMPLICATIONS ASSOCIATED WITH INFANTS OF DIABETIC MOTHERS

FETAL DEMISE
MACROSOMIA
RDS
WET LUNG SYNDROME (WITH CESAREAN)
HYPOGLYCEMIA
POLYCYTHEMIA
HYPOCALCEMIA
HYPERBILIRUBINEMIA
CONGENITAL MALFORMATIONS
Cardiac
Transposition of great vessels
Simple and complex ventricular
septal defect
Coarctation of the aorta
Central nervous system
Anencephaly
Holoprosencephaly
Meningomyelocele
Gastrointestinal
Anal/rectal atresia
Small left colon
Genitourinary
Renal agenesis
Ureteral duplication
Genital agenesis

Skeletal
Caudal regression
Femoral hypoplasia with unusual
facies syndrome
Vertebral anomalies
RENAL VEIN THROMBOSIS
CARDIOMYOPATHY
FAMILY PSYCHOLOGIC STRESS
(High risk pregnancy, fear of IDM)

Modified from: *Care of the High Risk Neonate*, Klaus MH, Fanaroff AA (eds), 3rd Edition, W.B. Saunders Company, Philadelphia, 1986, p.225.

RISK OF TRISOMY 21 BY MATERNAL AGE (AT DELIVERY)

AGE	RISK AT DELIVERY	RISK IN SECOND TRIMESTER
<20	1/1700	–
20-24	1/1350	–
25-29	1/1150	–
30	1/900	–
31	1/825	–
32	1/725	–
33	1/600	–
34	1/450	–
35	1/350	–
36	1/300	1/260
37	1/225	1/200
38	1/175	1/160
39	1/150	1/125
40	1/100	1/70
41	1/85	1/35
42	1/65	1/30
43	1/50	1/20
44	1/40	1/15
>45	1/25	1/10

Modified from: *The Science of and Practice of Pediatric Cardiology*, Gerson A Jr, Bricker JT, McNamara DG (eds), Lea & Febiger, Philadelphia, 1990, p.180.

MODIFIED WHITE'S CLASSIFICATION OF DIABETES IN PREGNANCY

CLASS A –	ABNORMAL GLUCOSE TOLERANCE TEST (GTT) WITH NORMAL FASTING BLOOD SUGAR (FBS); DIET CONTROL
CLASS B –	INSULIN-TREATED; ONSET AFTER 20 YEARS OF AGE; LESS THAN 10 YEARS' DURATION; NO VASCULAR DISEASE OR RETINOPATHY
CLASS C –	INSULIN-DEPENDENT; ONSET BETWEEN 10 AND 20 YEARS OF AGE; DURATION 10 TO 20 YEARS; NO VASCULAR DISEASE OR RETINOPATHY
CLASS D –	INSULIN-DEPENDENT; ONSET BEFORE 10 YEARS OF AGE; GREATER THAN 20 YEARS' DURATION; RETINOPATHY
CLASS F –	PREGNANT DIABETIC WITH DIABETIC NEPHROPATHY
CLASS G –	PREGNANT DIABETIC WITH PREVIOUS FETAL WASTAGE
CLASS H –	PREGNANT DIABETIC WITH CARDIOPATHY
CLASS R –	PREGNANT DIABETIC WITH MALIGNANT RETINOPATHY

Modified from: *Neonatology Pathophysiology and Management of the Newborn*, Avery GB (ed), 3rd Edition, J.B. Lippincott Company, Philadelphia, 1987, p.155.

RECURRENCE RISK OF COMMON BIRTH DEFECTS IN SUBSEQUENT PREGNANCIES

CHROMOSOMAL ABNORMALITY
Down syndrome (trisomy, 21) - 1%
SINGLE MUTANT GENE
Infantile polycystic kidney
disease - 25% (autosomal
recessive)
MULTIFACTORIAL INHERITANCE
Anencephaly - meningomyelocele - 2%
(alone or combined risk)
Ventricular septal defect - 4%
Cleft lip and palate - 4%
Cleft palate alone - 3%
Hypospadias - 7% of males
Club foot - 3%

Modified from: *Manual of Neonatal Care*, Cloherty JP, Stark AR (eds), 2nd Edition, Little Brown, Boston, 1985, p.129.

COMMON ABNORMALITIES IN THE ASPLENIC SYNDROME

ISOLATED LEVOCARDIA OR DEXTROCARDIA
VISCERAL ISOMERISM (MIDLINE LIVER AND
STOMACH)
TRANSPOSITION OF THE GREAT ARTERIES
DOUBLE OUTLET RIGHT VENTRICLE
TOTAL ANOMALOUS PULMONARY VENOUS RETURN
ENDOCARDIAL CUSHION DEFECT
PULMONARY ATRESIA OR STENOSIS
SINGLE VENTRICLE
BILATERAL SUPERIOR VENA CAVA
ABSENT CORONARY SINUS
IPSILATERAL INFERIOR VENA CAVA AND
ABDOMINAL AORTA
P-WAVE AXIS OF ATRIAL INVERSION
BILATERAL EPARTERIAL BRONCHI
BILATERAL TRILOBED LUNG

Modified from: *Neonatology Pathophysiology and Management of the Newborn*, Avery GB (ed), 3rd Edition, J.B. Lippincott Company, Philadelphia, 1987, p.521.

COMMON ABNORMALITIES IN THE POLYSPLENIA SYNDROME

DEXTROCARDIA OR LEVOCARDIA
ABSENT INFERIOR VENA CAVA (RENAL TO
    HEPATIC SEGMENT)
ENDOCARDIAL CUSHION DEFECT
TOTAL ANOMALOUS PULMONARY VENOUS RETURN
CORONARY SINUS RHYTHM
BILATERAL HYPARTERIAL BRONCHI

Modified from: *Neonatology Pathophysiology and Management of the Newborn*, Avery GB (ed), 3rd Edition, J.B. Lippincott Company, Philadelphia, 1987, p.155.

CAUSES OF MALE PSEUDOHERMAPHRODITISM

ABNORMAL GONADAL DIFFERENTIATION
    Mixed gonadal dysgenesis
    True hermaphroditism
ABNORMAL GONADAL FUNCTION
    Placental or fetal pituitary
        gonadotropin deficiency
    Leydig-cell agenesis
    Congenital anorchia (vanishing
        testes syndrome)
    Abnormalities of antimullerian
        hormone synthesis or action
DEFECTIVE TESTOSTERONE SYNTHESIS
ABNORMAL TESTOSTERONE METABOLISM
    5-Alpha-reductase deficiency
ABNORMAL TESTOSTERONE ACTION
    Testicular feminization (complete
        or incomplete)

Modified from: *Manual of Neonatal Care*, Cloherty JP, Stark AR (eds), 2nd Edition, Little Brown, Boston, 1985, p.373.

GENETICALLY DETERMINED DISEASES CAUSING HYPERAMMONEMIA

UREA CYCLE ENZYME DEFICIENCIES
Carbamyl phosphate synthetase
deficiency
Ornithine transcarbamylase
deficiency
Citrullinemia
Argininosuccinic acidemia
Argininemia (in some patients)
DISORDERS OF DIABASIC AMINO ACIDS
Ornithinemia
Periodic hyperlysinemia with
hyperammonemia
Persistent hyperlysinuria
Familial protein intolerance
DISORDERS OF BRANCHED-CHAIN AMINO ACIDS
B-ketothiolase deficiency
Propionicacidemias
Methylmalonicacidemias
Isovaleric acidemia
Glutaric acidemia II
Multiple carboxylase deficiency

Modified from: *Neonatology Pathophysiology and Management of the Newborn*, Avery GB (ed), 3rd Edition, J.B. Lippincott Company, Philadelphia, 1987, p.737.

CONDITIONS ASSOCIATED WITH DIARRHEA FROM TIME OF BIRTH

ABSORPTIVE DISORDERS (SYMPTOMS BROUGHT ON BY FEEDING)
    Glucose-galactose malabsorption
    Sucrase-isomaltase deficiency
    Lactase deficiency
    Cystic fibrosis
SECRETORY DISORDERS
    Congenital chloridorrhea
    Tumors
        Ganglioneuroma
        Neuroblastoma
OTHER
    Neonatal necrotizing enterocolitis
    Hirschsprung disease
    Intractable diarrhea of infancy
    Familial enteropathy

Modified from: *Schaffer's Diseases of the Newborn*, Avery ME, Taeusch HW (eds), 5th Edition, W.B. Saunders Company, Philadelphia, 1984, p.316.

CHAPTER XII

NEUROLOGY

CAUSES OF ACUTE ATAXIA

POST INFECTIOUS ACUTE CEREBELLAR ATAXIA
TOXINS
METABOLIC
- Hypoglycemia
- Hyponatremia
- Hyperammonemia
- Leigh disease

INFECTIONS
- Meningitis
- Encephalitis

WEAKNESS
- Guillain-Barré syndrome
- Myasthenic syndromes
- Tick paralysis

NEOPLASM
- Cerebellar tumor
- Brainstem glioma
- Neuroblastoma

HYDROCEPHALUS
STROKE
- Cerebellar hematoma infarct
- Brainstem hematoma infarct
- Cervical vertebral fracture
- Arteriovenous malformation
- Vasculitis
- Coagulopathy
- Sickle cell anemia
- Homocystinuria

VESTIBULAR DISTURBANCE
- Labyrinthitis
- Meniere disease
- Perilymphatic fistula

TRAUMA

Modified from: *Pediatric Neurology. Principles and Practice*, Swaiman KF (ed), C.V. Mosby Company, St. Louis, 1989, p.220.

Stumpf DA: *Pediatrics in Review* 8:303-306, 1987.

COMMON CAUSES OF VERTIGO IN CHILDREN

EAR DISORDERS
- Acoustic neuroma
- Acute otitis media
- Benign postural vertigo
- Chronic suppurative otitis media
- Endolymphatic hydrops
- Labyrinthitis
- Otic capsule fracture
- Ototoxicity (esp. aminoglycosides)
- Perilymphatic fistula
- Postmeningitis labyrinthitis
- Vestibular neuronitis

ASSOCIATED WITH CNS DISORDERS
- Demyelinating disease
- Neoplasm
- Posttraumatic
- Seizures
- Vestibulogenic migraine

ASSOCIATED WITH SYSTEMIC DISORDERS
- Hyperventilation
- Hypoglycemia
- Intoxication
- Psychogenic

Modified from: *The Whole Pediatrician Catalog*, McMillan JA, Stockman JA, Oski FA (eds), W.B. Saunders Company, Philadelphia, 1979, pp.276-277.

EXOGENOUS TOXINS CAUSING ACUTE ENCEPHALOPATHY

PHARMACOLOGIC AGENTS
- Sedative/hypnotics
- Narcotic analgesics
- Antihistamines
- Anticholinergics
- Anticonvulsants
- Phenothiazines
- Tricyclic antidepressants
- Salicylates
- Iron
- Penicillin
- Cimetidine
- Steroids

        DRUGS OF ABUSE
                Alcohol
                Amphetamines
                Narcotics
                Cannabis
                LSD
                Mescaline
                Psilocybin
                Phencyclidine
                Solvents
        ENVIRONMENTAL TOXINS
                Carbon monoxide
                Lead and heavy metals
                Organophosphates
                DDT
                Hydrocarbons
                Solvents

Modified from: *Principles and Practice of Pediatrics*, Oski FA, DeAngelis CD, Feigin RD, Warshaw JB (eds), J.B. Lippincott Company, Philadelphia, 1990, p.1847.

DRUGS THAT MAY INDUCE HALLUCINATIONS

        ALCOHOL
        AMPHETAMINES
        BELLADONNA
        COCAINE
        LSD
        MESCALINE
        PHENCYCLIDINE

Modified from: Felter R, Izsak E, Lawrence HS: *Pediatric Clinics of North America* 34:410, 1987.

DRUGS THAT MAY INDUCE SEIZURES

> CARBON MONOXIDE
> COCAINE
> CHLORINATED HYDROCARBONS
> DRUG WITHDRAWAL
> PCP
> PHENOTHIAZINES
> PROPROXYPHENE
> SYMPATHOMIMETICS

Modified from: Felter R, Izsak E, Lawrence HS: *Pediatric Clinics of North America* 34:410, 1987.

DRUGS AND TOXINS THAT MAY CAUSE DELIRIUM

> ALCOHOL
> AMINOPHYLLINE
> AMPHETAMINES
> ANTIHISTAMINES
> ATROPINE AND BELLADONNA
> BARBITURATES
> CAMPHOR
> CANNABIS
> CARBON MONOXIDE
> CIMETIDINE
> COCAINE
> ERGOT
> HYDROCARBONS
> LEAD AND OTHER HEAVY METALS
> LYSERGIC ACID
> MESCALINE
> OPIATES
> ORGANOPHOSPHATES
> PHENOTHIAZINES
> PROPRANOLOL
> SALICYLATES
> STRAMONIUM
> VERATRUM ALKALOIDS

Modified from: *Pediatric Neurology. Principles and Practice*, Swaiman KF (ed), C.V. Mosby Company, St. Louis, 1989, p.159.

DIFFERENTIAL DIAGNOSIS OF A PERSISTENTLY FLOPPY INFANT

CNS DISORDERS
>   Atonic diplegia
>   Congenital cerebellar ataxia
>   Kernicterus
>   Chromosomal defects
>   Lowe syndrome
>   Cerebral lipidoses
>   Prader-Willi syndrome

SPINAL CORD DISEASE
>   Trauma
>   Werdnig-Hoffman disease

DISEASES OF PERIPHERAL NERVE
>   Polyneuritis
>   Familial dysautonomia
>   Congenital sensory neuropathy

DISEASES OF NEUROMUSCULAR JUNCTION
>   Myasthenia gravis
>   Infantile botulism

MUSCLE DISEASES
>   Congenital muscular dystrophy
>   Myotonic dystrophy
>   Central core disease
>   Mitochondrial myopathies
>   Nemaline myopathy
>   Pompe disease

Modified from: *Nelson Textbook of Pediatrics*, Behrman R, Vaughan V (eds), W.B. Saunders Company, Philadelphia, 1987, p.1333.

CONDITIONS OFTEN ASSOCIATED WITH INFANTILE MYOCLONIC SPASMS

TUBEROUS SCLEROSIS
SPHINGOLIPIDOSES
PHENYLKETONURIA
MAPLE SYRUP DISEASE
AICARDI SYNDROME
ABSENCE OF CORPUS CALLOSUM
HOLOPROSENCEPHALY
HYPOGLYCEMIA
SUBDURAL HYGROMAS
HYDRANENCEPHALY
HYPOCALCEMIA
NONKETOTIC HYPERGLYCINEMIA
INTRAUTERINE INFECTION

DIFFERENTIAL DIAGNOSIS OF NEONATAL SEIZURES

AMINOACID DISTURBANCES
ASPHYXIA
CEREBRAL DYSGENESIS
DRUG WITHDRAWAL
    Barbiturate
    Heroin
    Methadone
    Propoxyphene
FAMILIAL SEIZURE DISORDERS
    Neonatal adrenoleukodystrophy
    Smith-Lemli-Opitz
    Incontinentia pigmenti
    Tuberous sclerosis
    Zellweger
    Benign familial epilepsy
INFECTIONS
    Bacterial meningitis
    Cerebral abscess
    Coxsackie meningoencephalitis
    Cytomegalovirus
    Herpes encephalitis
    Syphilis
    Toxoplasmosis
HYPERTENSION
METABOLIC
    Hypocalcemia
    Hypoglycemia
    Hyponatremia
    Hypernatremia
PYRIDOXINE DEPENDENCY
TOXINS
    Local anesthetics
    Isoniazid
    Bilirubin
TRAUMA
    Subdural hematoma
    Intracortical hemorrhage
    Cortical vein thrombosis

Modified from: *Pediatric Neurology. Principles and Practice*, Swaiman KF (ed), C.V. Mosby Company, St. Louis, 1989, p.429.

ETIOLOGY OF MACROCEPHALY

CONGENITAL
    Achondroplasia
    Benign familial
    Cranioskeletal dysplasia
    Craniosynostosis
    Hydranencephaly
    Hydrocephalus
    Megalencephaly
    Porencephaly
DEGENERATIVE
    Alexander disease
    Canavan spongy degeneration
INFECTIOUS
    Abscess
    Subdural effusion or empyema
METABOLIC
    Severe anemia
    Generalized gangliosidosis
    Maple syrup disease
    Metachromatic leukodystrophy
    Mucopolysaccharidoses
    Osteopetrosis
    Rickets
    Tay-Sachs disease
    Treatment of hypothyroidism
PSEUDOTUMOR CEREBRI
TRAUMATIC
    Leptomeningeal cyst
    Subdural hematoma or hygroma

Modified from: *Pediatric Neurology. Principles and Practice*, Swaiman KF (ed), C.V. Mosby Company, St. Louis, 1989, p.338.

DIFFERENTIAL DIAGNOSIS OF HYDROCEPHALUS

CONGENITAL
- Achondroplasia
- Agenesis of the corpus callosum
- Aqueductal stenosis
- Arachnoid cyst
- Arnold-Chiari malformation
- Basilar impression
- Dandy-Walker syndrome
- Encephalocele
- Osteopetrosis
- Porencephaly

DEGENERATIVE
- Incontinentia pigmenti
- Krabbe disease

INFECTIOUS
- Congenital syphilis
- Cytomegalic inclusion disease
- Mumps
- Postmeningitis
- Postencephalitis
- Toxoplasmosis

NEOPLASM
- Brainstem glioma
- Cerebellar astrocytoma
- Choroid plexus papilloma
- Colloid cyst of third ventricle
- Ependymoma
- Histiocytosis X
- Leukemia
- Lymphoma
- Medulloblastoma
- Neuroblastoma
- Pinealoma

TRAUMATIC
- Hemorrhage
- Ischemic encephalopathy
- Posterior fossa surgery

VASCULAR
- Arteriovenous malformation
- Jugular vein catheterization
- Vein of Galen malformation
- Venous sinus thrombosis

Modified from: *Pediatric Neurology. Principles and Practice*, Swaiman KF (ed), C.V. Mosby Company, St. Louis, 1989, p.338.

COMMON CAUSES OF HYDROCEPHALUS PRESENTING IN EARLY INFANCY

CONGENITAL
- Aqueductal stenosis
- Arnold-Chiari malformation
- Cranium bifidum
- Holoprosencephaly
- Spina bifida cystica
- INTRAUTERINE INFECTIONS
  - Cytomegalic inclusion disease
  - Rubella
  - Syphilis
  - Toxoplasmosis
- MASS LESIONS
  - A-V malformations
  - Congenital cysts
  - Neoplasms
- HEMORRHAGE
  - Hypoxia
  - Trauma
  - Vascular malformation
- PERI/POSTNATAL INFECTIONS
  - Bacterial
  - Granulomatous
  - Parasitic

CAUSES OF ENLARGED FONTANEL

ACHONDROPLASIA
ATHYROTIC HYPOTHYROIDISM
CLEIDOCRANIAL DYSOSTOSIS
DOWN SYNDROME
HYDROCEPHALUS
OSTEOGENESIS IMPERFECTA
RUBELLA SYNDROME
TRISOMIES 13 AND 18
AMINOPTERIN-INDUCED SYNDROME
APERT SYNDROME
HYPOPHOSPHATASIA
KENNY SYNDROME
PYKNODYSOSTOSIS
RICKETS
HALLERMANN-STREIFF SYNDROME
MALNUTRITION
PROGERIA
RUSSELL-SILVER SYNDROME

The Whole Pediatrician Catalog, McMillan JA, Nieburg PI, Oski FA (eds), W.B. Saunders Company, Philadelphia, 1977, p.4.

CAUSES OF A BULGING FONTANEL IN INFANCY

MENINGITIS
ENCEPHALITIS
HYDROCEPHALUS
CEREBRAL HEMORRHAGE
INTRACRANIAL ABSCESS
SUBDURAL HEMATOMA
LEAD POISONING
SINUS THROMBOSIS
TUMOR
BENIGN INTRACRANIAL HYPERTENSION

Modified from: *The Whole Pediatrician Catalog*, McMillan JA, Nieburg PI, Oski FA (eds), W.B. Saunders Company, Philadelphia, 1977, p.340.

CAUSES OF BENIGN INTRACRANIAL HYPERTENSION

ENDOCRINE/METABOLIC
    Addison disease
    Galactosemia
    Hypoparathyroidism
    Hypophosphatasia
    Hypothyroidism
DRUGS
    Hypervitaminosis A
    Tetracyclines
    Nalidixic acid
    Steroid therapy withdrawal
INFECTIONS
    Guillain-Barré syndrome
    Roseola infantum
    Otitis media
NUTRITIONAL
    Hypovitaminosis A
    Rapid brain growth following
      starvation
MISCELLANEOUS
    Allergic diseases
    Anemia
    Heart disease
    Polycythemia vera
    Wiskott-Aldrich syndrome
    Disseminated lupus
    Carbon dioxide retention secondary
      to chronic lung disease
    Sinus thrombosis

Modified from: *The Whole Pediatrician Catalog*,
McMillan JA, Nieburg PI, Oski FA (eds), W.B. Saunders
Company, Philadelphia, 1977, p.341.

DISEASES WITH INTRACRANIAL CALCIFICATION

ENDOCRINE
    Hypoparathyroidism
    Hyperparathyroidism
INFECTIOUS
    Brain abscess
    Cysticercosis
    Cytomegalic inclusion disease
    Toxoplasmosis
    Tuberculous meningitis

NEUROCUTANEOUS SYNDROMES
- Sturge-Weber
- Tuberous sclerosis

TUMORS
- Craniopharyngioma
- Ependymoma
- Oligodendroglioma
- Pinealoma
- Teratoma

VASCULAR
- Arteriovenous malformation
- Aneurysms

MISCELLANEOUS
- Fahr disease
- Idiopathic Basal ganglia calcification
- Lissencephaly
- Subdural hematoma (chronic)

Modified from: Babbitt DP, Tang T, Dobbs J, Berk R: *American Journal of Roentgenology* 105:356, 1969.

FINDINGS IN BASAL SKULL FRACTURE

BLEEDING FROM NOSE, EYES, OR EARS
DISCOLORATION IN THE MASTOID AREA
BLOOD BEHIND THE EARDRUM
CEREBROSPINAL RHINORRHEA
CRANIAL NERVE PALSIES (I, III, VIII)
SUBSEQUENT SINUSITIS
PNEUMOCEPHALY

Modified from: *The Best of The Whole Pediatrician Catalogs I-III*, McMillan JA, Oski FA, Stockman JA III, Nieburg PI (eds), W.B. Saunders Company, Philadelphia, p.386.

DIFFERENTIAL DIAGNOSIS OF CHRONIC AND RECURRENT HEADACHES IN CHILDHOOD

ANEURYSM
ARTERIOVENOUS MALFORMATION
BRAIN ABSCESS
BRAIN TUMOR
CHRONIC SUBDURAL HEMATOMA
CLUSTER
DENTAL PROBLEMS
EYE STRAIN
HYDROCEPHALUS
HYPOGLYCEMIA
MENINGEAL LEUKEMIA
MIGRAINE
NECK PROBLEMS
OCCIPITAL NEURALGIA
POST TRAUMATIC
PSEUDOTUMOR CEREBRI
PSYCHOGENIC
SEIZURE RELATED
SINUSITIS
TEMPOROMANDIBULAR JOINT SYNDROME
TENSION
TRIGEMINAL NEURALGIA

Modified from: Gascon GG: *Pediatric Clinics of North America* 31:1029-1030, 1984.

Olness KN, MacDonald JT: *Pediatrics in Review* 8:307-311, 1987.

CAUSES OF ACUTE PERIPHERAL CRANIAL NERVE VII PALSY

BELL PALSY
INFECTION
    Diphtheria
    Herpes zoster
    Mastoiditis
    Otitis media
    TB
GUILLAIN-BARRE SYNDROME

TRAUMA
    Basal skull fracture
    Post-surgical
    Penetrating trauma
TUMOR
    Brainstem
    Parotid
    Temporal bone
SARCOIDOSIS
CEREBROVASCULAR ACCIDENT

Modified from: Ohye RG, Altenberger EA: *American Family Practitioner* 40:159-65, 1989.

CHAPTER XIII

ONCOLOGY

CONDITIONS ASSOCIATED WITH ACUTE LEUKEMIA

FANCONI ANEMIA
BLOOMS ANEMIA
VON RECKLINGHAUSEN NEUROFIBROMATOSIS
CONGENITAL X-LINKED AGAMMAGLOBULINEMIA
ATAXIA-TELANGIECTASIA
SHWACHMAN SYNDROME
OSTEOGENESIS IMPERFECTA
MARFAN SYNDROME
KOSTMANN INFANTILE AGRANULOCYTOSIS
GLUTATHIONE REDUCTASE DEFICIENCY
ELLIS-VAN CREVELD SYNDROME
OSTEOCHONDROMATOSIS
ACHONDROPLASIA
HEREDITARY BRACHYDACTYLY, TYPE C
XERODERMA PIGMENTOSUM
INCONTINENTIA PIGMENTI
PHENYLKETONURIA
DOWN SYNDROME
IDENTICAL TWINS (UNDER 6 YEARS OF AGE)
  OF PATIENTS WITH ACUTE LEUKEMIA
D- AND F-TRISOMY
TURNER SYNDROME
XXY AND XYY CHROMOSOME DISORDERS
PARENTAL CONSANGUINITY
FAMILIAL LEUKEMIA
TREACHER COLLINS SYNDROME
RUBENSTEIN-TAYBI SYNDROME
POLAND SYNDROME
KLIPPEL-FEIL SYNDROME
BLACKFAN-DIAMOND SYNDROME
FAMILIAL CELLULAR FOLATE UPTAKE DEFECT
ATAXIA-PANCYTOPENIA
KLINEFELTER SYNDROME
WISKOTT-ALDRICH SYNDROME

Modified from: *Hematology of Infancy & Childhood*
Nathan DG, Oski FA (Eds), 3rd Edition, W.B. Saunders
Company, Philadelphia, 1987, p.925.

RELATIVE RISK OF LEUKEMIA IN SELECTED POPULATION GROUPS

POPULATION	RELATIVE RISK
Normal children	1.0
Siblings of leukemic child	1.1
Identical twin of leukemic child	350.0
Down syndrome	37.0
Fanconi anemia	1979.0
Bloom syndrome	2969.0
Ataxia telangiectasia	2969.0
Persons exposed to	
Atomic bomb, within 1000 m	47.0
Benzene	2.9
Alkylating agents	47.5

Modified from: *Blood Diseases of Infancy and Childhood*, Miller DR, Baehner RL (eds), 6th Edition, C.V. Mosby Company, St. Louis, 1989, p.607

MOST COMMON PRESENTATIONS OF ACUTE LYMPHOBLASTIC LEUKEMIA

LETHARGY/MALAISE
FEVER/INFECTION
BONE/JOINT PAIN
BLEEDING MANIFESTATION
ANOREXIA
ABDOMINAL PAIN
CNS MANIFESTATION
PALLOR

Modified from: *Hematology of Infancy & Childhood*, Nathan DG, Oski FA: H (eds), 3rd Edition, W.B. Saunders Company, Philadelphia, 1987, p.1036.

POOR PROGNOSTIC FACTORS IN ALL

WBC	>50,000/MM^3
AGE	<2 OR >10 YEARS
ORGAN INVOLVEMENT	++
THYMIC MASS	PRESENT
CNS INVOLVEMENT	PRESENT
CHROMOSOMAL TRANSLOCATION	PRESENT
SURFACE MARKERS	
T CELL	+
MATURE B CELL	+
CALLA+	−
UNDIFFERENTIATED	+

Modified from: *Hematology of Infancy & Childhood*,
Nathan DG, Oski FA (eds), 3rd Edition, W.B. Saunders
Company, Philadelphia, 1987, p.1048.

SIGNS AND SYMPTOMS OF CENTRAL NERVOUS SYSTEM LEUKEMIA

HEADACHES
VOMITING
LETHARGY
IRRITABILITY
SEIZURES
COMA
PAPILLEDEMA
DIPLOPIA
BLURRED VISION
PHOTOPHOBIA
BLINDNESS
NUCHAL RIGIDITY
HEMIPARESIS
PARAPLEGIA
SIXTH AND SEVENTH NERVE PALSIES
HYPERPHAGIA
SLEEP/WAKE DISTURBANCES
PATHOLOGIC WEIGHT GAIN
VERTIGO
AUDITORY DISTURBANCES
ATAXIA

HALLUCINATIONS
HYPERPNEA
PROPTOSIS
NYSTAGMUS
SLURRED SPEECH

Modified from: *Blood Diseases of Infancy and Childhood*,
Miller DR, Baehner RL (eds), 6th Edition, C.V. Mosby
Company, St. Louis, 1989, p.643

DISTRIBUTION OF GERM CELL TUMORS BY PRIMARY SITE

OVARY
SACROCOCCYGEAL REGION
TESTIS
INTRACRANIAL REGION
ABDOMEN/RETROPERITONEUM
MEDIASTINUM, HEART, LUNG
PHARYNX, NECK, THYROID
FEMALE GENITAL TRACT
SPINAL CORD, MENINGES
BLADDER, PROSTATE

Modified from: *Pediatrics*, Rudolph AM (ed), 18th
Edition, Appleton & Lange, Norwalk, 1987, p.1126.

CLINICAL MANIFESTATIONS OF HISTOCYTOSIS X

LETTERER-SIWE
Fever
Pulmonary interstitial infiltrate
Hepatosplenomegaly
Anemia
Thrombocytopenia
Lymphadenopathy
Skin rash
HAND-SCHULLER-CHRISTIAN
Lymphadenopathy
Skin rash
Exophthalmos
Diabetes insipidus
Otitis media
Growth retardation
Loss of dentition
Lytic bone lesion
SOLITARY EOSINOPHILIC GRANULOMA
Loss of dentition
Lytic bone lesion

Modified from: *Pediatrics*, Rudolph AM (ed), 18th
Edition, Appleton & Lange, Norwalk, 1987, p.1129.

CARCIONGENIC DRUGS

MEDICATIONS	ASSOCIATED NEOPLASMS
CHEMOTHERAPEUTIC AGENTS	
Busulfan	Acute leukemia
Chlorambucil	Acute leukemia
Cyclophosphamide	Acute leukemia, bladder cancer
Melphalan	Acute leukemia
Nitrosureas	Acute leukemia
HORMONES	
Androgenic steroids, oral contraceptives	Liver tumors
Estrogen compounds	Endometrial carcinoma
Prenatal diethylstilbestrol	Vaginal adenocarcinoma
RADIOISOTOPES	
Radioactive iodine	Thyroid cancer
Radium	Osteogenic sarcoma
Thorium dioxide	Liver tumors
MISCELLANEOUS	
Chloramphenicol	Acute leukemia
Immunosuppressives for organ transplantation	Lymphomas
Intramuscular iron	Sarcoma at injection site
Phenylbutazone	Leukemia
Prenatal hydantoin	Neuroblastoma

Modified from: *Hematology of Infancy & Childhood*, Nathan DG, Oski FA, (eds), 3rd Edition, W.B. Saunders Company, Philadelphia, 1987, p.923.

CHAPTER XIV

OPHTHALMOLOGY

CONDITIONS ASSOCIATED WITH CATARACTS

ALPORT SYNDROME
APERT SYNDROME
ATOPIC DERMATITIS
COCKAYNE SYNDROME
CONGENITAL ICHTHYOSIS
CONRADI SYNDROME
CROUZON DISEASE
DIABETES MELLITUS
ECTODERMAL DYSPLASIA
FABRY DISEASE
GALACTOSEMIA
HALLERMANN-STREIFF SYNDROME
HOMOCYSTINURIA
HYPOCALCEMIA
HYPOGLYCEMIA
HYPOPARATHYROIDISM
INCONTINENTIA PIGMENTI
INTRAUTERINE INFECTION
LAURENCE-MOON-BIEDL
LOWE SYNDROME
MARFAN SYNDROME
MARINESCO-SJOGREN SYNDROME
MYOTONIC DYSTROPHY
REFSUM DISEASE
ROTHMUND-THOMPSON SYNDROME
RUBENSTEIN-TAYBI SYNDROME
STICKLER SYNDROME
TRISOMY 13
TRISOMY 18
TRISOMY 21
TURNER SYNDROME
WILSON DISEASE

Modified from: *Ophthalmology - Principles and Concepts*, Newell FW (ed), 6th Edition, C.V. Mosby Company, St. Louis, 1986, p.368.

Pediatric Ophthalmology, Harley RD (ed), 2nd Edition, W.B. Saunders Company, Philadelphia, 1983, p.552-553.

DIFFERENTIAL DIAGNOSIS OF THE DISLOCATED LENS

CONGENITAL SYPHILIS
CROUZON DISEASE
EHLERS-DANLOS SYNDROME
HOMOCYSTINURIA
HYPERLYSINEMIA
MARFAN SYNDROME
SULFITE OXIDASE DEFICIENCY
TRAUMA
WEILL-MARCHESANI SYNDROME

Modified from: *Pediatric Ophthalmology*, Harley RD (ed),
2nd Edition, W.B. Saunders Company, Philadelphia, 1983,
p.301.

CONDITIONS ASSOCIATED WITH GLAUCOMA

ANIRIDIA
CHROMOSOMAL ABNORMALITIES
CONGENITAL RUBELLA
HOMOCYSTINURIA
LOWE SYNDROME
MARFAN SYNDROME
MUCOPOLYSACCHARIDOSIS
NEUROFIBROMATOSIS
PIERRE ROBIN SYNDROME
STURGE-WEBER SYNDROME
SECONDARY GLAUCOMA
        Intraocular tumors
        Retinopathy of prematurity
        Steroid induced
        Trauma

Modified from: *Ophthalmology - Principles and Concepts*,
Newell FW (ed), 6th Edition, C.V. Mosby Company, St. Louis,
1986, p.396.

CONDITIONS ASSOCIATED WITH BLUE SCLERA

ALBRIGHT HEREDITARY OSTEODYSTROPHY
CROUZON DISEASE
de LANGE SYNDROME
EHLERS-DANLOS SYNDROME
HALLERMANN-STREIFF SYNDROME

INCONTINENTIA PIGMENTI
IRON DEFICIENCY ANEMIA
MARFAN SYNDROME
MARSHALL-SMITH SYNDROME
OSTEOGENESIS IMPERFECTA
PSEUDOHYPOPARATHYROIDISM
PYKNODYSOSTOSIS
ROBERTS SYNDROME
RUSSELL-SILVER SYNDROME
TURNER SYNDROME

ETIOLOGY OF UVEITIS IN CHILDREN

ANKYLOSING SPONDYLITIS
BEHCET DISEASE
FUCHS HETEROCHROMIA
HERPES SIMPLEX
HISTOPLASMOSIS
PSORIASIS
REITER SYNDROME
SARCOIDOSIS
STILL DISEASE
SYMPATHETIC OPHTHALMIA
SYPHILIS
TOXOPLASMOSIS
TRAUMA
TUBERCULOSIS
ULCERATIVE COLITIS
VOGT-KOYANAGI-HARADA DISEASE

Modified from: *Pediatric Ophthalmology*, Harley RD (ed), 2nd Edition, W.B. Saunders Company, Philadelphia, 1983, p.519.

MORE COMMON CAUSES OF INFANTILE BLINDNESS

ALBINISM
"BATTERED BABY" RETINOPATHY
BILATERAL RETINOBLASTOMA
COLOBOMA OF MACULA
CONGENITAL CATARACTS
CONGENITAL GLAUCOMA

CONGENITAL HYDROCEPHALUS
LEBER'S CONGENITAL AMAUROSIS
OPTIC ATROPHY
OPTIC GLIOMA
RETINOPATHY OF PREMATURITY
TAY-SACHS DISEASE
TOXOPLASMOSIS

Modified from: Bancic JR: *Pediatric Clinics of North America*; 34:1405, 1987.

CAUSES OF PROPTOSIS IN CHILDREN

DYSOSTOSIS OF THE SKULL
MANDIBULOFACIAL DYSOSTOSIS
DEFECTS OF THE ORBITAL WALLS
    Encephalocele
    Meningocele
    Mucocele
DEVELOPMENTAL TUMORS
    Dermoid cyst
    Hemangioma
    Lipoma
    Lymphangioma
ORBITAL TUMORS
    Glioma
    Histiocytosis
    Leukemia
    Lymphoma
    Neuroblastoma
    Neurofibroma
    Pseudotumor
    Retinoblastoma
    Rhabdomyosarcoma
INFECTIOUS
    Orbital cellulitis
TRAUMA
    Orbital fracture
    Orbital hemorrhage
HYPERTHYROIDISM

Modified from: *Ophthalmology - Principles and Concepts*, Newell FW (ed), 6th Edition, C.V. Mosby Company, St. Louis, 1986, pp.268-271.

DIFFERENTIAL DIAGNOSIS OF OPTIC DISC EDEMA

OCULAR CONDITIONS
- Perforation of globe
- Generalized edema of ocular tissues
- Retinal vasculitis
- Neuroretinitis
- Uveitis

ORBITAL CONDITIONS
- Orbital tumor
- Abscess
- Aneurysm
- Nerve sheath hemorrhage
- Venous congestion
- Endocrine exophthalmos

INTRACRANIAL CONDITIONS
- Increased intracranial pressure
  - Intracranial tumor
  - Hydrocephalus
  - Brain abscess
  - Encephalitis, meningitis
  - Encephalopathy
  - Intracracranial hemorrhage
  - Dural sinus thrombosis
  - Pseudotumor cerebri
- Decreased intracranial space
- CSF protein elevation

SYSTEMIC CONDITIONS
- Hypertension
- Blood dyscrasia
  - Anemias
  - Leukemias
  - Thrombocytopenia
  - Polycythemia
  - Macroglobulinemia
- Cardiopulmonary disorders
  - Congestive heart failure
  - Cystic fibrosis
  - Pickwickian syndrome

ENDOCRINE DISORDER
- Hyperthyroidism
- Hypoparathyroidism
- Addison disease
- Juvenile diabetes mellitus

COLLAGEN VASCULAR DISEASES

Modified from: *Pediatric Ophthalmology*, Harley RD (ed), 2nd Edition, W.B. Saunders Company, Philadelphia, 1983, p.815.

CHAPTER XV

ORTHOPEDICS

RECOMMENDATIONS FOR PARTICIPATION IN COMPETITIVE SPORTS

CONTACT/COLLISION SPORTS
- Boxing
- Field hockey
- Football
- Ice hockey
- Lacrosse
- Martial arts
- Rodeo
- Soccer
- Wrestling

LIMITED CONTACT/IMPACT SPORTS
- Baseball
- Basketball
- Bicycling
- Diving
- Gymnastics
- High jump
- Horseback riding
- Pole vault
- Skating
  - Ice
  - Roller
- Skiing
  - Cross-country
  - Downhill
  - Water
- Softball
- Squash, handball, raquetball
- Volleyball

STRENUOUS NONCONTACT SPORTS
- Aerobic dancing
- Crew
- Fencing
- Field
  - Discus
  - Javelin
  - Shotput
- Running
- Swimming
- Tennis
- Track
- Weight lifting

CONDITION FOR WHICH ONLY CONTACT SPORTS
ARE CONTRAINDICATED
Absence of one kidney

CONDITIONS FOR WHICH CONTACT AND LIMITED
CONTACT SPORTS ARE CONTRAINDICATED
Atlantoaxial instability *
Enlarged liver
Poorly controlled convulsive disorder **

CONDITIONS FOR WHICH CONTACT SPORTS AND
STRENUOUS NONCONTACT SPORTS ARE
CONTRAINDICATED
Enlarged spleen
Mitral valve prolapse ***

CONDITION FOR WHICH ALL SPORTS ACTIVITY IS
CONTRAINDICATED
Carditis

*   No swimming (butterfly stroke, breast
        stroke, or diving starts)
**   No swimming, weightlifting, archery, and
        riflery
***   If any history of syncope, family
        history of sudden death due to mitral
        valve prolapse, chest pain worsened by
        exercise, repetitive forms of
        ventricular ectopic activity, moderate
        or marked mitral regurgitation,
        associated dilation of the ascending
        aorta, or associated Marfan syndrome.
        Patients without these findings may
        engage in all competitive sports.

Modified from: Committee on Sports Medicine: *Pediatrics*
81:737-739, 1988.

DISORDERS ASSOCIATED WITH SCOLIOSIS

CONGENITAL
IDIOPATHIC
TUMORS
    Osteoid osteoma
    Osteoblastoma
    Intraspinal
TRAUMA
    Vertebral trauma
    Post-irradiation
NEUROMUSCULAR
    Cerebral palsy
    Poliomyelitis
    Meningomyelocele
    Syringomyelia
    Friedreich ataxia
    Familial dysautonomia
    Hypertrophic interstitial
      polyneuritis
    Peroneal muscular atrophy
    Juvenile spinal muscle atrophy
    Duchenne muscular dystrophy
    Limb-girdle muscular dystrophy
    Arthrogryposis
MISCELLANEOUS
    Achondroplasia
    Chondrodysplasia punctata
    Cornelia deLange
    Cri du Chat
    Cystic fibrosis
    Diastrophic dwarfism
    Down
    Ehlers-Danlos
    Juvenile rheumatoid arthritis
    Klippel-Feil
    Laurence-Moon-Biedl
    Leg length discrepancy
    Maple syrup urine disease
    Marfan
    Metatropic dwarfism
    Mucopolysaccharidoses
    Neurofibromatosis
    Osteogenesis imperfecta
    Prader-Willi
    Rickets
    Rubinstein-Taybi
    Scheuermann deformity

Spondyloepiphyseal dysplasia
  congenita
Turner syndrome
Upper limb amelia

Modified from: Rothner DA: *J Pediatr* 86:748-750, 1975.

Diagnosis of Bone and Joint Disorders, Resnick D,
Niwayama G (eds), 2nd Edition, W.B. Saunders Company,
Philadelphia, 1988, p.3526.

DIFFERENTIAL DIAGNOSIS OF TORTICOLLIS

CONGENITAL
  Transient postural torticollis
  C_1-C_2 articular malformation
  Klippel-Feil syndrome
  Sprengel deformity
  Muscular torticollis
TRAUMA TO VERTEBRAE OR CLAVICLE
INFECTION
  Pharyngitis
  Retropharyngeal abscess
  Cervical adenopathy
TUMORS
  Posterior fossa
  Intraspinal
  Osteoid osteoma
  Eosinophilic granuloma
NEUROLOGIC
  Dystonia
  Syringomyelia
  Herniated cervical disks
  Poliomyelitis
  Huntington chorea
  Wilson disease
  Kernicterous
  Spastic torticollis
MISCELLANEOUS
  Drugs (especially phenothiazines)
  Sandifer syndrome
  Ocular strabismus
  Paroxysmal torticollis

Modified from: Bredenkamp JK, Hoover LA, Berke GS, Shaw A:
Arch Otolaryngology Head Neck Surgery 116:213, 1990.

Clark RN: *Pediatric Annals* 5:43, 1976.

DISORDERS ASSOCIATED WITH SLIPPED CAPITAL FEMORAL EPIPHYSIS

ACROMEGALY
CRANIOPHARYNGIOMA
GIGANTISM
GROWTH HORMONE THERAPY
HYPERPARATHYROIDISM
HYPOGONADISM
HYPOPITUITARISM
HYPOTHYROIDISM
KLINEFELTER SYNDROME
MARFAN SYNDROME
RADIATION THERAPY
RENAL OSTEODYSTROPHY

Modified from: *Diagnosis of Bone and Joint Disorders*, Resnick D, Niwayama G (eds), 2nd Edition, W.B. Saunders Company, Philadelphia, 1988, pp.2962-2965.

Pediatric Orthopedics, Tachdjian MO (ed), 2nd Edition, W.B. Saunders Company, Philadelphia, 1990, p.1016.

DISORDERS ASSOCIATED WITH OSTEOPOROSIS

IDIOPATHIC JUVENILE OSTEOPOROSIS
IMMOBILIZATION
ENDOCRINE
    Hyperthyroidism
    Hyperparathyroidism
    Cushing
    Acromegaly
    Diabetes mellitus
    Hypogonadism
    Pregnancy or lactation
SEVERE ANEMIA
OSTEOGENESIS IMPERFECTA
COLLAGEN-VASCULAR
    Ankylosing spondylitis
    Juvenile rheumatoid arthritis

DRUG INDUCED
    Steroids
    Heparin
DEFICIENCY STATES
    Calcium deficiency
    Copper deficiency
    Protein-calorie malnutrition
    Scurvy
METABOLIC
    Gaucher
    Niemann-Pick
    Fabry
    Homocystinuria
    Hyperphosphatasia
MISCELLANEOUS
    Familial Mediterranean fever
    Hemochromatosis
    Congenital cutis laxa with osteoporosis
    Osteoporosis with pseudogliomatous
      blindness

Modified from: *Diagnosis of Bone and Joint Disorders,*
Resnick D, Niwayama G (eds), 2nd Edition, W.B. Saunders
Company, Philadelphia, 1988, p.2025.

DIFFERENTIAL DIAGNOSIS OF CHILDHOOD BACK PAIN

POSTURAL PROBLEMS
MUSCLE STRAIN
SCHEUERMANN KYPHOSIS
SPONDYLOLYSIS/SPONDYLOLISTHESIS
HERNIATED NUCLEUS PULPOSUS
FRACTURE OF VERTEBRAL BODY
DISCITIS
BACTERIAL OSTEOMYELITIS (INCLUDING POTT
  DISEASE)
COLLAGEN VASCULAR DISORDER
NEOPLASTIC DISEASES
    Osteoid osteoma
    Osteoblastoma/osteosarcoma
    Leukemia/lymphoma
    Eosinophilic granuloma
    Ewing sarcoma
    Neuroblastoma
    Spinal cord tumor

Modified from: King JA: *Pediatric Clinics of North
America* 33:1491, 1986.

DIFFERENTIAL DIAGNOSIS OF ARTHRALGIA

INFECTION-RELATED DISORDERS
- Septic arthritis
- Osteomyelitis
- Mycoplasma
- Tuberculosis
- Syphilis
- Viral infections
  - Parvovirus
  - Infectious mononucleosis
  - Rubella
  - Mumps
  - Hepatitis B
  - Arbovirus
  - Adenovirus
- Enteric bacterial infections
  - Shigella
  - Salmonella
  - Campylobacter
  - Yersinia
- Lyme disease

MALIGNANCY
- Leukemia/lymphoma
- Neuroblastoma
- Bone tumors

RHEUMATIC AND INFLAMMATORY DISEASES
- Acute rheumatic fever
- Juvenile rheumatoid arthritis
- Systemic lupus erythematosus
- Dermatomyositis
- Scleroderma
- Mixed connective tissue diseases
- Juvenile ankylosing spondylitis
- Psoriatic spondyloarthritis
- Reiter disease
- Kawasaki syndrome
- Serum sickness
- Henoch-Schönlein purpura
- Inflammatory bowel disease
- Subacute bacterial endocarditis

ORTHOPEDIC CONDITIONS
    Trauma related
    Mechanical derangement
    Chondromalacia of patella
    Legg-Calvé-Perthes disease
    Osgood-Schlatter disease
    Slipped capital femoral epiphysis
    Osteochondritis diseases
    Blount disease
MISCELLANEOUS
    Toxic synovitis
    Vitamin A poisoning
    Rickets
    Marfan syndrome
    Hemoglobinopathy
    Hypermobility syndrome
    Postimmunization (MMR)
    Psychosomatic complaints
    Referred pain
    Familial Mediterranean fever
    Amyloidosis
    Gout
    Sarcoidosis
    Lysosomal storage diseases
    Reflex neurovascular dystrophy

Modified from: *Differential Diagnosis in Pediatrics*, Stockman JA III (ed), W.B. Saunders Company, Philadelphia, 1990, p.338.

CAUSES OF HEMIHYPERTROPHY

NEUROCUTANEOUS SYNDROMES
      Neurofibromatosis
      Tuberous sclerosis
      Sturge-Weber disease
      Lindau-von Hippel disease
SKIN AND VASCULAR ABNORMALITIES
      Angiodysplasias
      Lymphatic abnormalities
      Lipomatosis
TUMORS
      Wilms
      Adrenocortical tumors
      Hepatoblastoma
RENAL ABNORMALITIES
      Nephromegaly
      Medullary sponge kidney
DYSMORPHOGENIC SYNDROMES
      Russell-Silver
      Beckwith-Wiedemann
      Langer-Giedion
      Proteus

Modified from: *Diagnosis of Bone and Joint Disorders*, Resnick D, Niwayama G (eds), 2nd Edition, W.B. Saunders Company, Philadelphia, 1988, p.4276.

Signs and Symptoms in Pediatrics, Tunnessen WW (ed), 2nd Edition, J.B. Lippincott, Philadelphia, 1988, p.510.

DISEASES ASSOCIATED WITH CALF HYPERTROPHY

DUCHENNE MUSCULAR DYSTROPHY
X-LINKED MUSCULAR DYSTROPHY
AUTOSOMAL RECESSIVE PSEUDOHYPERTROPHIC
  MUSCULAR DYSTROPHY
LIMB-GIRDLE MUSCULAR DYSTROPHY
HYPERKALEMIC PERIODIC PARALYSIS
LATE INFANTILE ACID MALTASE DEFICIENCY
PHOSPHOGLUCOMUTASE DEFICIENCY

Modified from: *Signs and Symptoms in Pediatrics*,
Tunnessen WW (ed), 2nd Edition, J.B. Lippincott,
Philadelphia, 1988, p. 527.

DISORDERS ASSOCIATED WITH ATLANTOAXIAL
  INSTABILITY

DOWN SYNDROME
RHEUMATOID ARTHRITIS
ANKYLOSING SPONDYLITIS
PSORIATIC ARTHRITIS
REITER SYNDROME
DYGGRE-MELCHIOR-CLAUSEN DYSPLASIA
GRISEL SYNDROME
HURLER SYNDROME
MARFAN SYNDROME
METAPHYSICAL CHONDRODYSPLASIA
METATROPIC DYSPLASIA
MORQUIO SYNDROME
MULTICENTRIC RETICULOHISTIOCYTOSIS
NEUROFIBROMATOSIS
PSEUDOACHONDROPLASIA
SPONDYLOEPIPHYSEAL DYSPLASIA CONGENITA
TUBERCULOUS SPONDYLITIS
BEHCET SYNDROME
REGIONAL ENTERITIS

Modified from: *Diagnosis of Bone and Joint Disorders*,
Resnick D, Niwayama G (eds), 2nd Edition, W.B. Saunders
Company, Philadelphia, 1988.

CHAPTER XVI

OTOLARYNGOLOGY

ETIOLOGY OF NECK MASSES

CYSTIC
     Branchial cleft cyst
     Cystic hygroma
     Thyroglossal duct cyst
SOLID
     Infectious lymphadenopathy
     Lymphoma
     Metastatic lymph nodes
     Neurogenic tumors
     Carotid body tumors
     Thyroid masses

Modified from: *Fundamentals of Otolaryngology. A Textbook of Ear, Nose, and Throat Diseases*, Adams GL, Boies LR Jr, Hilger PA (eds), 6th Edition, W.B. Saunders Company, Philadelphia, 1989, p.433.

COMMON AGENTS PRODUCING ESOPHAGEAL BURNS

AMMONIA
BLEACH
CLINITEST TABLETS
DRAIN CLEANERS (NAOH)
IODINE
NITRIC ACIDS
OVEN CLEANERS
PHENOL
PHOSPHATES
POTASSIUM PERMANGANATE
SULFURIC ACIDS

Modified from: *Fundamentals of Otolaryngology. A Textbook of Ear, Nose, and Throat Diseases*, Adams GL, Boies LR Jr, Hilger PA (eds), 6th Edition, W.B. Saunders Company, Philadelphia, 1989, p.473.

FOODS MOST COMMONLY CAUSING ASPHYXIATION IN CHILDREN

> HOT DOGS
> CANDY
> PEANUTS
> GRAPES
> COOKIES
> BISCUITS
> MEAT

Modified from: Stockman JA III: *Journal Club Newsletter*
5:1, 1990.

ABSOLUTE INDICATIONS FOR TONSILLECTOMY/ ADENOIDECTOMY

> DEVELOPMENT OF COR PULMONALE
> ASSOCIATED SLEEP APNEA
> DYSPHAGIA WITH ASSOCIATED WEIGHT LOSS
> SUSPECTED MALIGNANCY
> RECURRENT PERITONSILLAR ABSCESS

Modified from: *Fundamentals of Otolaryngology. A Textbook
of Ear, Nose, and Throat Diseases*, Adams GL, Boies LR Jr,
Hilger PA (eds), 6th Edition, W.B. Saunders Company,
Philadelphia, 1989, p.352.

MAJOR CAUSES OF SENSORINEURAL HEARING LOSS

> DIABETES
> HYPERLIPOPROTEINEMIAS
> OTOSCLEROSIS
> Rh INCOMPATIBILITY
> PAGET DISEASE
> RETINITIS PIGMENTOSA
> RUBELLA
> PENDRED DISEASE (NONENDEMIC GOITER)

Modified from: *Fundamentals of Otolaryngology. A
Textbook of Ear, Nose, and Throat Diseases*, Adams GL,
Boies LR Jr, Hilger PA (eds), 6th Edition, W.B. Saunders
Company, Philadelphia, 1989, p.127.

INDICATIONS FOR AUDIOLOGIC EVALUATION

BIRTH WEIGHT < 2500 g: ALL CASES
BIRTH WEIGHT > 2500 g: WITH FOLLOWING
  COMPLICATIONS
      Asphyxia
      Assisted ventilation
      Hyperbilirubinemia
      Intracranial hemorrhage
      Ototoxic drugs
      Persistent fetal circulation
      Seizures
BACTERIAL MENINGITIS
PROVEN OR SUSPECTED INTRAUTERINE
  INFECTION
ANOMALIES OF 1st OR 2nd BRANCHIAL ARCH
ANOMALIES OF NEURAL CREST/ECTODERM
FAMILY HISTORY OF HEREDITARY OR
  UNEXPLAINED DEAFNESS
PARENTAL CONCERN REGARDING HEARING LOSS
DELAYED SPEECH OR LANGUAGE DEVELOPMENT
OTHER DEVELOPMENTAL DISABILITIES
      Autism
      Blindness
      Cerebral palsy
      Mental retardation

Modified from:*Difficult Diagnosis in Pediatrics*,
Stockman JA III (ed), W.B. Saunders Company, Philadelphia,
1990, p.34.

CONDITIONS ASSOCIATED WITH NASAL POLYPS

ALLERGIES
ASPIRIN SENSITIVITY
ASTHMA
CHRONIC NASAL INFECTION
CYSTIC FIBROSIS
MALIGNANCY
SINUSITIS

Modified from: *Nose and Sinus Surgery*, Balkany TJ,
Pashley NRT (eds), C.V. Mosby, St. Louis, 1986, p.318.

Ear, Nose and Throat Disorders in Children, Bordley
JE, Brookhouser PE, Tucker GF Jr (eds), Raven Press
Books, New York City, 1986, p.254.

CAUSES OF A PERFORATED NASAL SEPTUM

TRAUMA
Nose picking
Operative procedures
SYPHILIS
TUBERCULOSIS
WEGENER GRANULOMATOSIS
CARCINOMA
COCAINE ADDICTION
INHALATION OF ACID FUMES
LEPROSY

Modified from: *Fundamentals of Otolaryngology. A Textbook of Ear, Nose, and Throat Diseases*, Adams GL, Boies LR Jr, Hilger PA (eds), 6th Edition, W.B. Saunders Company, Philadelphia, 1989, p.246.

Textbook of Otolaryngology, DeWeese DD, Saunders WH (eds), C.V. Mosby Company, St. Louis, 1982, p. 201.

CAUSES OF EPISTAXIS

COMMON
Environmental
Dry air
Nasal irritants
Sudden barometric changes
Foreign body
Rhinitis
Sinusitis
Trauma
External blunt trauma
Nose picking
Upper respiratory infection
UNCOMMON
Drug effects
Anticoagulants
Aspirin
Decongestant abuse
Hematologic
Coagulopathy
Platelet dysfunction
Sickle cell anemia
Thrombocytopenia

Hypertension
Idiopathic
Infectious
    Congenital syphilis
    Nasal diphtheria
    Rheumatic fever
    Scarlet fever
    Tuberculosis
    Typhoid fever
Postoperative
Structural
    Nasal polyps
    Nasal septal deviations
    Nasal septal perforation
Tumors
    Angiofibroma
    Angioma
    Granuloma
    Papilloma
Vascular anomalies
    Hemangioma
    Osler-Weber-Rendu

Modified from: *Nose and Sinus Surgery*, Balkany TJ, Pashley NRT (eds), C.V. Mosby, St. Louis, 1986, p.297-298.

Principles and Practice of Pediatrics, Oski FA, DeAngelis CD, Feigin RD, Warshaw JB (eds), J.B. Lippincott, Philadelphia, 1990, p.2033.

OTOTOXIC DRUGS

ANALGESICS
  Salicylates
ANTIBIOTICS
  Aminoglycosides
  Chloramphenicol
  Chloroquine
  Colistin
  Erythromycin
  Pharmacetin
  Polymyxin B
  Quinine
  Ristocetin
  Vancomycin
ANTINEOPLASTIC
  Bleomycin
  Cisplatin
  Nitrogen mustard
DIURETICS
  Acetazolamide
  Ethacrynic acid
  Furosemide
  Mannitol
MISCELLANEOUS
  Hexadine
  Mandelamine
  Pentobarbital
  Practolol

Modified from: *Fundamentals of Otolaryngology. A Textbook of Ear, Nose, and Throat Diseases*, Adams GL, Boies LR Jr, Hilger PA (eds), 6th Edition, W.B. Saunders Company, Philadelphia, 1989, p.132.

MAJOR COMPLICATIONS OF SINUSITIS

ORBITAL
    Cellulitis (orbital, periorbital,
      or preseptal)
    Orbital abscess
    Optic neuritis
    Subperiosteal abscess
OSTEOMYELITIS
    Frontal
    Maxillary
INTRACRANIAL
    Brain abscess
    Cavernous or sagittal sinus
      thrombosis
    Epidural abscess
    Meningitis
    Subdural empyema or abscess

Modified from: *Principles and Practice of
Pediatrics*, Oski FA, DeAngelis CD, Feigin RD, Warshaw
JB (eds), J.B. Lippincott, Philadelphia, 1990, p.882.

FACTORS PREDISPOSING TO SINUS OSTIAL
OBSTRUCTION

SYSTEMIC DISORDER
    Allergic inflammation
    Cystic fibrosis
    Immotile cilia
    Immune disorders
    Viral URI
LOCAL INSULT
    Facial trauma
    Rhinitis medicamentosa
    Swimming, diving
STRUCTURAL ABNORMALITIES
    Choanal atresia
    Deviated septum
    Foreign body
    Nasal polyps
    Tumor

Modified from: *Principles and Practice of
Pediatrics*, Oski FA, DeAngelis CD, Feigin RD, Warshaw
JB (eds), J.B. Lippincott, Philadelphia, 1990, p.879.

CHAPTER XVII

PULMONOLOGY

DIFFERENTIAL DIAGNOSIS OF WHEEZING

ASTHMA
BRONCHIOLITIS
BRONCHOPULMONARY DYSPLASIA
CYSTIC FIBROSIS
GE REFLUX WITH ASPIRATION
FOREIGN BODY ASPIRATION
TRACHEOBRONCHOMALACIA
IMMUNODEFICIENCY SYNDROMES
TUBERCULOSIS
VASCULAR RING
TRACHEOESOPHAGEAL FISTULA
IDIOPATHIC PULMONARY HEMOSIDEROSIS
CARDIAC DISEASE
MEDIASTINAL MASS
ALLERGIC BRONCHOPULMONARY ASPERGILLOSIS
ALPHA-1-ANTITRYPSIN DEFICIENCY
PARASITIC PNEUMONIAS
SARCOIDOSIS

Modified from: Goldenhush MJ, Rachelesfsky GS:
Pediatrics in Review 10:227-233,1989.

Nickerson BG: *Pediatric Annals* 15:99-104, 1986.

CONDITIONS ASSOCIATED WITH PULSUS PARADOXUS

CONGESTIVE HEART FAILURE
CARDIAC TAMPONADE
ASTHMA
CYSTIC FIBROSIS
BRONCHIOLITIS

Modified from: *The History and Physical Examination*, Kendig EL, Chernick V (eds), 4th Edition, W.B. Saunders Company, Philadelphia, 1983, p.65.

CAUSES OF STRIDOR IN THE NEONATE

CONGENITAL CYSTS
LARYNGEAL WEB
LARYNGOMALACIA
SUBGLOTTIC STENOSIS
TRACHEOMALACIA
VASCULAR ANOMALIES
VOCAL CORD PARALYSIS
HYPOCALCEMIA

Modified from: *The Pediatric Chest*, Felman AH (ed),
Charles C Thomas Publisher, Springfield, 1983, pp.404-410.

CAUSES OF STRIDOR IN CHILDHOOD

ALLERGIC REACTION
ASPIRATION OF FOREIGN BODIES
CROUP
EPIGLOTTITIS
PERITONSILLAR ABSCESS
RETROPHARYNGEAL ABSCESS
SUBGLOTTIC STENOSIS
TONSIL/ADENOID HYPERTROPHY

Modified from: *The Pediatric Chest*, Felman AH (ed),
Charles C Thomas Publisher, Springfield, 1983, pp. 410-432.

TUMORS OF THE ANTERIOR MEDIASTINUM

LYMPHOMA
THYMOMA
TERATODERMOID
INTRATHORACIC GOITOR
ANGIOMATOUS TUMOR

Modified from: *Pulmonary Medicine*, Guenter CA, Welch MH
(eds), 2nd Edition, J.B. Lippincott Company, Philadelphia,
1982, p.884.

TUMORS OF THE MIDDLE MEDIASTINUM

> LYMPHADENOPATHY
> LYMPHOMA
> METASTATIC CARCINOMA
> SARCOIDOSIS
> INFECTIOUS GRANULOMA
> BRONCHOGENIC AND ENTERIC CYSTS
> HIATAL HERNIA
> ANEURYSM
> PERICARDIAL CYST

Modified from: *Pulmonary Medicine*, Guenter CA, Welch MH (eds), 2nd Edition, J.B. Lippincott Company, Philadelphia, 1982, p.884.

Brecher ML: *J Respiratory Disease* 7:73-87, 1986.

TUMORS OF THE POSTERIOR MEDIASTINUM

> NEUROGENIC TUMOR
> AORTIC ANEURYSM
> INFECTIOUS SPONDYLITIS
> MENINGOCELE
> PHEOCHROMOCYTOMA
> DIAPHRAGMATIC HERNIA
> HEMANGIOMA
> DUPLICATION CYST

Modified from: *Pulmonary Medicine*, Guenter CA, Welch MH (eds), 2nd Edition, J.B. Lippincott Company, Philadelphia, 1982, p. 884.

Brecher ML: *J Respiratory Disease* 7:73-87, 1986.

DISEASES ASSOCIATED WITH CLUBBING

> BILIARY ATRESIA
> BILIARY CIRRHOSIS
> BRONCHIECTASIS
> CHRONIC DYSENTERY
> CHRONIC PNEUMONIAS
> CHRONIC ULCERATIVE COLITIS
> CONGENITAL CYANOTIC HEART DISEASE

CYSTIC FIBROSIS
EMPYEMA
FAMILIAL (BENIGN)
HIV INFECTION
INTERSTITIAL FIBROSIS
POLYPOSIS
PULMONARY ABSCESS
PULMONARY NEOPLASMS
REGIONAL ENTERITIS
SUBACUTE BACTERIAL ENDOCARDITIS
THYROTOXICOSIS

Modified from: *Disorders of the Respiratory Tract in
Children*, Kendig EL, Chernick V (eds), 4th edition, W.B.
Saunders Company, Philadelphia, 1983, p.68.

CONDITIONS ASSOCIATED WITH HEMOPTYSIS

TRAUMA
COAGULOPATHY
INFECTIONS
    Bronchitis/Bronchiectasis
    Pneumonias
        Bacterial
        Fungal
        Parasitic
        Tuberculosis
    Lung abscess
    Intracavitary fungus balls
NEOPLASMS
    Bronchial adenomas
    Bronchogenic cancer
    Endobronchial metastases
    Tracheal tumors
VASCULAR DISORDERS
    Arteriovenous malformations
    Cardiac failure with pulmonary edema
    Mitral stenosis
    Pulmonary embolism and infarction
VASCULITIC DISORDERS
    Systemic lupus erythematosus
    Wegener granulomatosis

MISCELLANEOUS
    Cystic fibrosis
    Goodpasture syndrome
    Heiner syndrome (cow's milk
        sensitivity)
    Idiopathic pulmonary hemosiderosis
    Pulmonary sequestration

Modified from: *Allergic Diseases from Infancy to
Adulthood*, Bierman CW, Pearlman DS (eds), 2nd
Edition, W.B. Saunders Company, Philadelphia, 1988,
p.628.

CAUSES OF CHRONIC COUGH

INFECTION
    Pneumonia
    Pharyngitis
    Laryngitis
    Sinusitis
    Pertussis
    Parapertussis
    Influenza
    Tuberculosis
    Spasmodic croup
TRAUMA
    Foreign body
INFLAMMATORY
    Asthma
    Allergic/Post-nasal drip
PHYSICAL CHEMICAL IRRITANTS
    Smoke (Tobacco/Firewood)
    Dry, dusty environment
    Volatile chemicals (hydrocarbons)
    Aspiration
CONGENITAL
    Tracheoesophageal fistula
    Vascular ring
    Laryngomalacia
    Laryngeal cysts
    Bronchogenic cysts
    Pulmonary sequestration
    Immotile cilia syndrome
PSYCHOGENIC/HABIT

MISCELLANEOUS
>   Cystic Fibrosis
>   Congestive heart failure
>   Gastroesophageal reflux
>   Bronchopulmonary dysplasia
>   Mediastinal mass

Modified from: Morgan WJ, Taussig LM: *Pediatrics in Review* 8:249-253, 1987.

Wilmott RW: *Contemporary Pediatrics* 4:26-43, 1987.

CONDITIONS ASSOCIATED WITH PNEUMOTHORACES

FIRST BREATH
IATROGENIC
>   Mechanical ventilation
>   Thoracentesis
>   Lung/Pleural biopsy
>   Cardiothoracic surgery
>   Cardiopulmonary resuscitation
LOWER RESPIRATORY TRACT DISEASES
>   Aspiration
>   Asthma
>   Bronchiolitis
>   Cystic fibrosis
>   Hyaline membrane disease
>   Malignancy
>   Pneumonia
TRAUMA

Modified from: *Disorders of the Respiratory Tract in Children*, Kendig EL, Chernick V (eds), 4th edition, W.B. Saunders Company, Philadelphia, 1983, p.492.

SPECIFIC ETIOLOGIES OF PLEURAL EFFUSIONS

TRANSUDATES
- Cardiovascular
  - Congestive heart failure
  - Constrictive pericarditis
  - Superior vena caval obstruction
- Increased extracellular fluid volume
  - Hypoalbuminemia
  - Salt-retaining syndromes
- Intra-abdominal process
  - Cirrhosis with ascites
  - Peritoneal dialysis

EXUDATES
- Infections
  - Bacterial empyema
  - Fungi
  - Parasites
  - Tuberculosis
  - Viruses
- Trauma
  - Hemothorax
  - Chylothorax
  - Esophageal rupture
- Neoplasm
  - Bronchogenic carcinoma
  - Metastatic carcinoma
  - Lymphoma
  - Mesothelioma
  - Intra-abdominal tumors
- Connective tissue diseases
  - Lupus erythematosus
  - Rheumatoid arthritis
- Intra-abdominal diseases
  - Pancreatitis
  - Subdiaphragmatic abscess
  - Abdominal surgery
  - Hepatitis
- Idiopathic

Miscellaneous
        Pulmonary embolus
        Post-myocardial infarction syndrome
        Lymphedema
        Familial Mediterranean fever
        Myxedema

Modified from: *Pulmonary Medicine*, Guenter CA, Welch MH
(eds), 2nd Edition, J.B. Lippincott Company, Philadelphia,
1982, p.578.

ETIOLOGIC FACTORS IN BRONCHIECTASIS

        IDIOPATHIC
        DEFECTS OF CILIA
        CYSTIC FIBROSIS
        IMMUNOLOGIC DEFICIENCY
        INFECTION
        OBSTRUCTION
        ATELECTASIS
        CORROSIVE GASES

Modified from: *Pulmonary Medicine*, Guenter CA, Welch MH
(eds), 2nd Edition, J.B. Lippincott Company, Philadelphia,
1982, p.747.

MANIFESTATIONS OF CYSTIC FIBROSIS

NASAL POLYPOSIS
SINUSITIS
ALLERGIC BRONCHOPULMONARY ASPERGILLOSIS
ATELECTASIS
BRONCHIECTASIS
BRONCHIOLITIS
BRONCHITIS
COR PULMONALE
HEMOPTYSIS
PNEUMOTHORAX
PNEUMONIA
REACTIVE AIRWAY DISEASE
RESPIRATORY FAILURE
CHOLECYSTITIS
CHOLELITHIASIS
CHOLESTASIS
CIRRHOSIS
PORTAL HYPERTENSION
ARTHROPATHY
ABSENT VAS DEFERENS
ASPERMIA
DECREASED FEMALE FERTILITY
DELAYED PUBERTY
DIGITAL CLUBBING
ERYTHEMA NODOSUM
FAILURE TO THRIVE
GROWTH RETARDATION
MALNUTRITION
GASTROESOPHAGEAL REFLUX
INTUSSUSCEPTION
MECONIUM ILEUS
MECONIUM ILEUS EQUIVALENT
MECONIUM PLUG SYNDROME
PANCREATIC EXOCRINE DEFICIENCY
PANCREATITIS
PEPTIC ULCER DISEASE
RECTAL PROLAPSE
DIABETES
HYPOKALEMIC ALKALOSIS
HYPOPROTHROMBINEMIA
IRON DEFICIENCY ANEMIA
SALT DEPLETION SYNDROME

PROTEIN-CALORIE MALNUTRITION
VITAMIN A DEFICIENCY
VITAMIN E DEFICIENCY

Modified from: *Principles and Practice of Pediatrics*,
Oski FA, DeAngelis CD, Feigin RD, Warshaw JB (eds), J.B.
Lippincott Company, Philadelphia, 1990, p.554.

ETIOLOGY OF CHRONIC INTERSTITIAL LUNG DISEASE

ALVEOLAR PROTEINOSIS
ASPIRATION PNEUMONITIS
BRONCHIOLITIS OBLITERANS
CYSTIC FIBROSIS
GAUCHER DISEASE
GOODPASTURE SYNDROME
HISTIOCYTOSIS X
HYPERSENSITIVITY PNEUMONITIS
IDIOPATHIC INTERSTITIAL PNEUMONITIS
INFECTIONS
NEUROFIBROMATOSIS
NIEMANN-PICK DISEASE
PULMONARY HEMOSIDEROSIS
RADIATION PNEUMONITIS
SARCOIDOSIS
TRACHEOESOPHAGEAL AND GREAT VESSEL
  MALFORMATIONS
TUBEROUS SCLEROSIS
VASCULITIS
WEGENER GRANULOMATOSIS

Modified from: *Difficult Diagnosis in Pediatrics*,
Stockman JA III (ed), W.B. Saunders, Company, Philadelphia,
1990, p.365.

CONDITIONS ASSOCIATED WITH PERSISTENT PULMONARY INFILTRATES

BRONCHIAL ADENOMA
BRONCHOPULMONARY DYSPLASIA
BRONCHOGENIC CYST
CONGENITAL LOBAR EMPHYSEMA
DRUG TOXICITY
FOREIGN BODY ASPIRATION
HISTIOCYTOSIS
HYDROCARBON ASPIRATION
PULMONARY ALVEOLAR PROTEINOSIS
PULMONARY SEQUESTRATION
RADIATION TOXICITY
SARCOIDOSIS
TUBERCULOSIS
WEGENER GRANULOMATOSIS

Modified from: *Difficult Diagnosis in Pediatrics*, Stockman JA III (ed), W.B. Saunders, Company, Philadelphia, 1990, p.376.

CONDITIONS ASSOCIATED WITH RECURRENT PULMONARY INFILTRATES

ACQUIRED IMMUNODEFICIENCY SYNDROME
ASTHMA
CHRONIC GRANULOMATOUS DISEASE
CYSTIC FIBROSIS
GASTROESOPHAGEAL REFLUX
GOODPASTURE SYNDROME
HEINER SYNDROME
H-TYPE TRACHEOESOPHAGEAL FISTULA
HYPERSENSITIVITY PNEUMONITIS
HYPOGAMMAGLOBULINEMIA
IDIOPATHIC PULMONARY HEMOSIDEROSIS
IMMOTILE CILIA SYNDROME
RECURRENT ASPIRATION SECONDARY TO
    NEUROLOGIC DISEASE
VASCULAR RING

Modified from: *Difficult Diagnosis in Pediatrics*, Stockman JA III (ed), W.B. Saunders, Company, Philadelphia, 1990, p.376.

CONDITIONS ASSOCIATED WITH ADULT RESPIRATORY DISTRESS SYNDROME

SEPSIS
SHOCK
ASPIRATION
NEAR DROWNING
TRAUMA
PNEUMONIA
TOXIC GAS INHALATION
DRUG POISONING

Modified from: *The Lung, Normal and Diseased*, Whitcomb ME, C.V. Mosby Company, St. Louis, 1982, p.279.

PNEUMOCONIOSES AND RELATED INDUSTRIAL TRADES

CONDITIONS	INDUSTRIAL TRADES
ALUMINUM PNEUMOCONIOSIS	FIREWORKS MANUFACTURING
ASBESTOSIS	AUTO MECHANICS
	CARPENTRY
	MILL WORKERS
	MINERS
BARITOSIS	BARITE MINER
	CERAMICS WORKER
	PAINT MANUFACTURING
BERYLLIOSIS	CERAMICS WORKER
	FLUORESCENT LAMP
	MANUFACTURING
COAL MINER'S PNEUMOCONIOSIS	COAL MINING
SIDEROSIS	FLAME CUTTER
	FOUNDRY WORKER
	WELDER
SILICOSIS	BRICKLAYER
	CERAMICS WORKER
	COAL MINER
	SANDBLASTER
	STONE CUTTER
TALCOSIS	CERAMICS WORKER
	COSMETICS WORKER
	MINER
	PLASTICS WORKER
	RUBBER WORKER

Modified from: *Pulmonary Medicine*, Guenter CA, Welch MH (eds), 2nd Edition, J.B. Lippincott Company, Philadelphia, 1982, pp.638-648.

CHAPTER XVIII

TOXICOLOGY/PHARMACOLOGY

FREQUENTLY INGESTED PRODUCTS THAT ARE USUALLY NONTOXIC

ANTACIDS
BABY PRODUCT COSMETICS
BALL-POINT INKS
BATH OIL (CASTOR OIL AND PERFUME)
BATTERY (DRY CELL)
BLEACH (LESS THAN 6% SODIUM
  HYPOCHLORITE)
BUBBLE BATH SOAPS
CALAMINE LOTION
CANDLES
CHALK
CLAY (MODELING)
CRAYONS (MARKED A,P,CP OR CS)
DEHUMIDIFYING PACKETS
DETERGENTS (PHOSPHATE ONLY)
ELMERS GLUE
EYE MAKEUP
FISH BOWL ADDITIVES
GOLF BALL (MAY CAUSE MECHANICAL INJURY)
HAND LOTIONS & CREAMS
HYDROGEN PEROXIDE (MEDICINAL 3%)
INK (BLACK, BLUE [NON-PERMANENT])
LIPSTICK
MINERAL OIL (UNLESS ASPIRATED)
NEWSPAPER (CHRONIC MAY RESULT IN LEAD
  POISONING)
PENCILS (LEAD AND COLORING)
PLAY-DOH
PUTTY AND SILLY PUTTY
SACHETS
SHAMPOO
SHAVING CREAMS AND LOTIONS
SOAP
SHOE POLISH (OCCASIONALLY ANILINE DYES
  PRESENT)
SWEETENING AGENTS (SACCHARIN, CYCLAMATE)
TEETHING RINGS
THERMOMETERS
TOOTHPASTE
VASELINE
WATER COLORS
ZINC OXIDE

TREATMENT NECESSARY ONLY IF INGESTED IN
  LARGE AMOUNTS
    After shave lotion
    Cologne
    Deodorant

Fabric softeners
Hair products (dyes, sprays, tonics)
Indelible markers
Matches
No Doz
Oral contraceptives
Perfume
Suntan preparations
Toilet water

Modified from: *The Best of the Whole Pediatrician
Catalogs I-III*, McMillan JA, Oski FA, Stockman JA III,
Nieburg PI (eds), W.B. Saunders Company, Philadelphia, 1984,
p.496.

Handbook of Common Poisonings in Children, Aronow R
(ed), 2nd Edition, American Academy of Pediatrics, Evanston,
1983, p.18.

POISONS ASSOCIATED WITH COMA

AMPHETAMINES
ANTICHOLINERGIES
BARBITURATES
CARBAMAZEPINE
CARBON MONOXIDE
CHLORAL HYDRATE
COCAINE
ETHANOL
ISOPROPYL ALCOHOL
HALOPERIDOL
NARCOTICS
PHENCYCLIDINE (PCP)
PHENOTHIAZINES
PHENYTOIN
SALICYLATES
SEDATIVE/HYPNOTICS
TRICYCLIC ANTIDEPRESSANTS

Modified from: *Emergency Pediatrics*, Barkin RM, Rosen P
(eds), C.V. Mosby Company, St. Louis, 1990, p.288.

COMMON NONTOXIC PLANTS

ABELIA
AFRICAN DAISY
AFRICAN PALM
AFRICAN VIOLET
AIRPLANE PLANT
ALUMINUM PLANT
ARALIA
ASPARAGUS FERN
  (MAY CAUSE
  DERMATITIS)
ASPIDISTRA (CAST
  IRON PLANT)
ASTER
BABY'S TEARS
BACHELOR BUTTONS
BEGONIA
BIRDS NEST FERN
BLOOD LEAF PLANT
BOSTON FERNS
BOUGAINVILLEA
CACTUS - CERTAIN
  VARIETIES
CALIFORNIA HOLLY
CALIFORNIA POPPY
CAMELIA
CHRISTMAS CACTUS
COLEUS
CORN PLANT
CRAB APPLES
CREEPING CHARLIE
CREEPING JENNIE,
  MONEYWORT,
  LYSIMA
CROTON (HOUSE
  VARIETY)
DAHLIA
DAISIES
DANDELION
DOGWOOD
DONKEY TAIL

DRACAENA
EASTER LILY
ECHEVERIA
EUGENIA
GARDENIA
GRAPE IVY
HEDGE APPLES
HENS & CHICKS
HONEYSUCKLE
HOYA
IMPATIENS
JADE PLANT
KALANCHOE
LILY (DAY, EASTER
  OR TIGER)
LIPSTICK PLANT
MAGNOLIA
MARIGOLD
MONKEY PLANT
MOTHER-IN-LAW
  TONGUE
NORFOLK ISLAND PINE
PEPEROMIA
PETUNIA
PRAYER PLANT
PURPLE PASSION
PYRACANTHA
ROSE
SANSEVIERIA
SCHEFFLERA
SENSITIVE PLANT
SPIDER PLANT
SWEDISH IVY
UMBRELLA
VIOLETS
WANDERING JEW
WEEPING FIG
WEEPING WILLOW
WILD ONION
ZEBRA PLANT

Modified from: *Textbook of Pediatric Emergency Medicine*, Fleisher G, Ludwig S (eds), 2nd Edition, Williams & Wilkins, Baltimore, 1988, p. 595.

COMMON PLANT TOXIDROMES

GASTROINTESTINAL IRRITANTS
- Philodendron
- Diffenbachia
- Pokeweed
- Wisteria
- Spurge laurel
- Buttercup
- Daffodil
- Rosary pea
- Castor bean

DIGITALIS EFFECTS
- Lily-of-the-valley
- Foxglove
- Oleander

NICOTINIC EFFECTS
- Wild tobacco
- Golden chain tree
- Poison hemlock

ATROPINIC EFFECTS
- Jimsonweed (thorn apple)

EPILEPTOGENIC EFFECTS
- Water hemlock

CYANOGENIC EFFECTS
- Prunus species (chokecherry, wild black cherry, plum, peach, apricot, bitter almond)
- Pear (seeds)
- Apple (seeds)
- Crab apple (seeds)
- Hydrangea
- Elderberry

Modified from: *Emergency Pediatrics*, Barkin RM, Rosen P (eds), C.V. Mosby Company, St. Louis, 1990, p.594.

CLASSIFICATION OF HYDROCARBONS

NONTOXIC (UNLESS COMPLICATED BY GROSS ASPIRATION)
- Asphalt
- Tars
- Mineral oil
- Liquid petrolatum
- Motor oil
- Axle grease
- Baby oil
- Suntan oil

SYSTEMIC TOXICITY
- Halogenated
  - Carbon tetrachloride
  - Trichloroethane
- Aromatic
  - Benzene
  - Toluene
  - Xylene
- Additives
  - Camphor
  - Organophosphates
  - Heavy metals

ASPIRATION HAZARD (SIGNIFICANT SYSTEMIC TOXICITY ONLY IF INGESTED IN MASSIVE QUANTITY)
- Turpentine
- Gasoline
- Kerosene
- Mineral seal oil
- Charcoal lighter fluid
- Cigarette lighter fluid
- Mineral spirits

Modified from: *Emergency Pediatrics*, Barkin RM, Rosen P (eds), C.V. Mosby Company, St. Louis, 1990, p.586.

TOXIDROMES

ANTICHOLINERGICS
- Vital signs (VS)
  - Fever
  - Tachycardia
  - Hypertension
  - Cardiac arrythmias (TCA)
- Central nervous system signs (CNS)
  - Delirium
  - Psychosis
  - Convulsions
  - Coma
- Eye
  - Mydriasis
- Skin
  - Flushed
  - Hot
  - Dry

AMPHETAMINES
    Vital signs
        Fever
        Tachycardia
        Hypertension
    Central nervous system signs
        Hyperactive to delirious
        Tremor
        Myoclonus
        Psychosis
        Convulsions
    Eye
        Mydriasis
    Skin
        Sweaty
NARCOTICS
    Vital signs
        Bradycardia
        Bradypnea
        Hypotension
        Hypothermia
    Central nervous system signs
        Euphoria to coma
        Hyporeflexia
    Eye
        Pinpoint pupils
ORGANOPHOSPHATES
    Vital signs
        Bradycardia
        Tachypnea
    Central nervous system signs
        Confusion to drowsiness to coma
        Convulsions
        Fasciculations
        Weakness to paralysis
    Eye
        Miosis
        Blurry vision
        Lacrimation
    Skin
        Sweaty
    Odor
        Garlic
    Other
        Salivation
        Bronchorrhea
        Bronchospasm
        Pulmonary edema
        Urinary frequency
        Diarrhea

BARBITURATES, SEDATIVES AND HYPNOTICS
Vital signs
Hypothermia
Hypotension
Bradypnea
Central nervous system signs
Confusion to coma
Ataxia
Eye
Nystagmus
Miosis to mydriasis
Skin
Vesicles
Bullae
SALICYLATES
Vital signs
Fever
Hyperpnea
Central nervous system signs
Lethargy to coma
Odor
Oil of wintergreen
(methylsalicylate)
Other
Vomiting
PHENOTHIAZINES
Vital signs
Postural hypotension
Hypothermia
Tachycardia
Tachypnea
Central nervous system signs
Lethargy to coma
Tremor
Convulsions
Ataxia
Torticollis
Back arching
Oculogyric crisis
Trismus
Tongue protrusion or heaviness
Eye
Miosis (majority)

THEOPHYLLINE
    Vital signs
        Tachycardia
        Hypotension
        Cardiac arrhythmias
        Tachypnea
    Central nervous system signs
        Agitation
        Convulsions
    Other
        Vomiting

Modified from: *Emergency Pediatrics*, Barkin RM, Rosen P (eds), C.V. Mosby Company, St. Louis, 1990, p.558.

HYDROCARBONS IN ORDER OF INCREASING VOLATILITY (THERFORE INCREASING RISK OF ASPIRATION WITH INGESTION)

    TAR
    PARAFFIN WAX
    LUBRICATING OIL
    FUEL OIL
    MINERAL SEED OIL
    KEROSENE
    MINERAL SPIRITS
    GASOLINE
    PETROLEUM NAPHTHA
    PETROLEUM ETHER

Modified from: Klein BL, Simon JE: *Pediatric Clinics of North America* 33:412, 1986.

BREATH ODOR AND ASSOCIATED POISONINGS

ACRID (PEAR-LIKE)
    Paraldehyde
ALCOHOL
    Ethanol
    Chloral hydrate
    Phenols
ACETONE
    Acetone
    Salicylates
    Isopropyl alcohol
    Chloroform
    Lacquer
    Ketoacidosis
BITTER ALMONDS
    Cyanide (in chokecherry, apricot
        pits)
BURNED ROPE
    Marijuana
COAL GAS (STOVE GAS)
    Carbon monoxide
GARLIC
    Arsenic
    Phosphorus
    Organophosphates
PUNGENT, AROMATIC
    Ethchlorvynol (Placidyl)
ROTTEN EGGS
    Hydrogen sulfide mercaptans
SHOE POLISH
    Nitrobenzene
STALE TOBACCO
    Nicotine
VIOLETS
    Turpentine
WINTERGREEN
    Methylsalicylate

Modified from: *The Best of the Whole Pediatrician Catalogs I-III*, McMillan JA, Oski FA, Stockman JA III, Nieburg PI (eds), W.B. Saunders Company, Philadelphia, 1984, p.506.

Emergency Pediatrics, Barkin RM, Rosen P (eds), C.V. Mosby Company, St. Louis, 1990, p.295.

RADIOPAQUE MEDICATIONS AND CHEMICALS

    CHLORAL HYDRATE
    HEAVY METALS (ARSENIC, LEAD)
    IRON
    IODIDES
    PHENOTHIAZINES
    PSYCHOTROPICS (TCA)
    ENTERIC COATED TABLETS
    SLOW-RELEASE CAPSULES

Modified from: *Emergency Pediatrics*, Barkin RM, Rosen P
(eds), C.V. Mosby Company, St. Louis, 1990, p.295.

FERRIC CHLORIDE TEST (URINE AND SERUM)

CONDITION OR DRUG	COLOR
PHENYLKETONURIA	BLUE-GREEN
HISTIDINEMIA	BLUE-GREEN
BILIRUBIN	BLUE-GREEN
TYROSINEMIA	BLUE-GREEN (TRANSIENT)
MAPLE SYRUP URINE DISEASE	GREENISH GRAY
KETOSIS	REDDISH BROWN
PYRUVIC ACID	DEEP YELLOW
XANTHURENIC ACID	DARK GREEN
MELANIN	GRAY PRECIPITATE
SALICYLATES	PURPLE
PHENOTHIAZINES	GREEN
LYSOL INGESTION	GREEN
NORMAL URINE	BROWN-WHITE

Modified from: *The Best of the Whole Pediatrician
Catalogs I-III*, McMillan JA, Oski FA, Stockman JA III,
Nieburg PI (eds), W.B. Saunders Company, Philadelphia, 1984,
p.500.

CONTRAINDICATIONS FOR INDUCING EMESIS

> DECREASED LEVEL OF CONSCIOUSNESS
> INGESTED MATERIAL LIKELY TO CAUSE RAPID
>   ONSET OF NEUROLOGIC SYMPTOMS
> CONVULSIONS
> STRONG CAUSTIC MATERIAL (ACID OR ALKALI)
>   INGESTION
> ABSENT GAG REFLEX

Modified from: *Textbook of Pediatric Emergency Medicine*, Fleisher G, Ludwig S (eds), 2nd Edition, Williams & Wilkins, Baltimore, 1988, p.550.

Rodgers GC, Matyunas NJ: *Pediatric Clinics of North America* 33:261-285, 1986.

RELATIVE CONTRAINDICATIONS FOR INDUCING EMESIS

> VERY YOUNG (LESS THAN 6 MONTHS OF AGE)
> INGESTION OF MOST HYDROCARBONS
> LATE-STAGE PREGNANCY
> SEVERE CARDIAC OR RESPIRATORY DISEASE
> UNCONTROLLED HYPERTENSION

Modified from: *Textbook of Pediatric Emergency Medicine*, Fleisher G, Ludwig S (eds), 2nd Edition, Williams & Wilkins, Baltimore, 1988, p.550.

Rodgers GC, Matyunas NJ: *Pediatric Clinics of North America* 33:261-285, 1986.

SUBSTANCES WELL ABSORBED BY ACTIVATED CHARCOAL

ACETAMINOPHEN
AMINOPHYLLIN
AMPHETAMINES
ANTIMONY
ANTIPYRENE
ARSENIC
ASPIRIN
ATROPINE
BARBITURATES
BENZODIAZEPINES
CANTHARIDES
COCAINE
DDT (CHLORINATED
   HYDROCARBONS)
DIGITALIS
DILANTIN
GLUTETHIMIDE
IODINE
IPECAC
MALATHION
MEPROBAMATE
MERCURIC CHLORIDE
METHYLENE BLUE

MORPHINE
MUSCARINE
NICOTINE
OPIUM
OXALATES
PARATHION
   (ORGANOPHOSPHATES)
PENICILLIN
PHENOL
PHENOLPHTHALEIN
PHENOTHIAZINES
PHOSPHORUS
POTASSIUM PERMANGANATE
PROPOXYPHENE
QUININE
SELENIUM
SILVER
STRAMONIUM
STRYCHNINE
SULFONAMIDES
TRICYCLIC ANTI-
   DEPRESSANTS

Modified from: *Textbook of Pediatric Emergency Medicine*, Fleisher G, Ludwig S (eds), 2nd Edition, Williams & Wilkins, Baltimore, 1988, p.551.

Albert S: *Pediatric Clinics of North America* 34:61-71, 1987.

SUBSTANCES POORLY (OR NOT) ABSORBED BY ACTIVATED CHARCOAL

COMMON ELECTROLYTES
IRON
MINERAL ACIDS OR BASES
ALCOHOLS
CYANIDE
MOST SOLVENTS
MOST WATER-INSOLUBLE COMPOUNDS

Modified from: *Textbook of Pediatric Emergency Medicine*, Fleisher G, Ludwig S (eds), 2nd Edition, Williams & Wilkins, Baltimore, 1988, p.551.

RENAL EXCRETION OF FREQUENTLY USED DRUGS

GLOMERULAR FILTRATION
    Aminoglycosides
    Vancomycin
    Digoxin
    Flucytosine
TUBULAR SECRETION
    Organic Acids
        Penicillins
        Cephalosporins
        Furosemide
        Thiazide diuretics
        Methotrexate
    Organic Bases
        Procainamide
        Triamterene

ENHANCED METHODS OF RENAL DRUG EXCRETION

ALKALINE DIURESIS
    Salicylate
    Phenobarbital
ACID DIURESIS
    Amphetamine
    Chloroquine
    Lidocaine
NEUTRAL DIURESIS
    Aliphatic alcohols
    Meprobamate
    Lithium

Modified from: Peterson RG, Peterson LN: *Pediatric Clinics of North America* 33:687, 1986.

DRUGS AND THEIR PLASMA CONCENTRATIONS FOR WHICH HEMODIALYSIS SHOULD BE CONSIDERED

LITHIUM	4.0 mEq/L
ETHYLENE GLYCOL	50 mg/dl
METHANOL	50 mg/dl
SALICYLATES	100 mg/dl

Modified from: *Textbook of Pediatric Emergency Medicine*, Fleisher G, Ludwig S (eds), 2nd Edition, Williams & Wilkins, Baltimore, 1988, p.556.

DRUGS AND THEIR PLASMA CONCENTRATIONS FOR WHICH HEMOPERFUSION SHOULD BE CONSIDERED

PHENOBARBITAL	100 mg/dl
OTHER BARBITURATES	5 mg/dl
THEOPHYLLINE	60-100 mg/L
PARAQUET	0.1 mg/dl
GLUTETHIMIDE	4 mg/dl
METHAQUALONE	4 mg/dl
ETHCHLORVYNOL	15 mg/dl
MEPROBAMATE	10 mg/dl

Modified from: *Textbook of Pediatric Emergency Medicine*, Fleisher G, Ludwig S (eds), 2nd Edition, Williams & Wilkins, Baltimore, 1988, p.556.

APPROXIMATE VOLUMES OF DISTRIBUTION IN L PER KG

ACEBUTOLOL	1.2
ACETAMINOPHEN	1.0
AMINOGLYCOSIDES	0.2-0.5
AMOBARBITAL	1.1
AMPHETAMINE	0.6
AMPHOTERICIN B	4.0
BENZODIAZEPINES	3.0-10.0
CAFFEINE	0.9
CARBAMAZEPINE	1.4
CHLORAMPHENICOL	0.9
CIMETIDINE	2.1
DIGOXIN	7.5

FUROSEMIDE	0.2
INDOMETHACIN	0.9
LITHIUM	0.8
LOCAL ANESTHETICS	1.0-1.5
NARCOTICS	3.0-5.0
PENICILLINS	0.2-0.3
PENTOBARBITAL	1.0
PHENOBARBITAL	0.75 (1.0)*
PHENOTHIAZINES	20.0-30.0
PHENYTOIN	0.75 (1.0)*
PREDNISONE	1.0
PROPRANOLOL	4.0
QUINIDINE	3.0
SALICYLATE	0.2 (THERAPEUTIC DOSES)
	0.6 (TOXIC DOSES)
SECOBARBITAL	1.5
THEOPHYLLINE	0.46 (0.69)
TRICYCLIC ANTI-DEPRESSANTS	8.0-30.0
VALPROIC ACID	0.1

* Values in parentheses are for newborns

Modified from: Peterson RG, Peterson LN: *Pediatric Clinics of North America* 33:678, 1986.

COMMON SOURCES OF LEAD

LOW DOSE
    Food
    Ambient air
    Drinking water
INTERMEDIATE DOSE
    Dust (household)
    Interior lead paint removal
    Contaminated soil (automobile
      exhaust)
    Industrial sources
    Improper removal of exterior lead
      paint
HIGH DOSE
    Interior and exterior lead paint

Modified from: American Academy of Pediatrics Committee on Environmental Hazards and Committee on Accident and Poison Prevention: *Pediatrics* 79:457-465, 1987.

UNCOMMON SOURCES OF LEAD

METALLIC OBJECTS (SHOT, FISHING WEIGHT)
LEAD GLAZED CERAMICS
OLD TOYS AND FURNITURE
STORAGE BATTERY CASINGS
GASOLINE SNIFFING
LEAD PLUMBING
EXPOSED LEAD SOLDER IN CANS
IMPORTED CANNED FOODS AND TOYS
FOLK MEDICINES
    Mexican
        Azarcon
        Greta
    Chinese
        Pay-loo-ah
LEADED GLASS ARTWORK
COSMETICS
    Ceruse
    Surma
    Kohl
ANTIQUE PEWTER
FARM EQUIPMENT

Modified from: American Academy of Pediatrics Committee on
Environmental Hazards and Committee on Accident and Poison
Prevention: *Pediatrics* 79:457-465, 1987.

AGENTS THAT MAY AFFECT THE FETUS ADVERSELY

ALCOHOL
ANTINEOPLASTIC DRUGS
AMINOPTEXIN
ANDROGENS
    Methyltestosterone
AZATHIOPRINE
CHLOROQUINE
COUMARIN
CYCLOPHOSPHAMIDE
DIETHYLSTILBESTROL (DES)
DIPHENYLHYDANTOIN
HERBICIDES
IODIDES
LITHIUM CARBONATE

MEPIVACAINE
METHIMAZOLE
METHOTREXATE
METHYLMERCURY
NONPRESCRIPTION DRUGS
    Aspirin (heavy use)
    Caffeine (heavy use)
    Smoking - Nicotine
    Vitamins
        A (massive doses)
        D (massive doses)
OXAZOLIDINE - 2,4 DIONES
    Paramethadione
    Trimethadione
PENICILLAMINE
PHENYTOIN (DILANTIN)
POLYCHLORINATED BIPHENYLS
PROGESTINS
    Norlutin
PROPRANOLOL
PROPYLTHIOURACIL
QUININE
RADIATION
RADIOIODINE
STREET DRUGS
STREPTOMYCIN
TETRACYCLINE
THALIDOMIDE
TOLBUTAMIDE
VALPROATE

Modified from: *Assessment and Care of the Fetus. Physiological, Clinical, and Medicolegal Principles*, Eden RD, Boehm FH, Haire M (eds), Appleton & Lange, Norwalk, 1990, pp.223-244.

Nelson Textbook of Pediatrics. Nelson WE, Behrman RE, Vaughan VC III (eds), 13th Edition, W.B. Saunders Company, Philadelphia, 1987, pp.370-371.

TRADITIONAL CLASSIFICATION OF BARBITURATES

LONG ACTING
    Mephobarbital
    Metharbital
    Phenobarbital
SHORT-TO-INTERMEDIATE ACTING
    Amobarbital
    Butabarbital
    Pentobarbital
    Secobarbital
ULTRASHORT ACTING
    Hexobarbital
    Methohexital
    Thiopental

Modified from: Bertino JS, Reed MD: *Pediatric Clinics of North America* 33:705, 1986.

RADIOPHARMACEUTICALS THAT REQUIRE TEMPORARY CESSATION OF BREAST-FEEDING

GALLIUM-67
    (Radioactivity in milk present
     for 2 weeks)
INDIUM-111
    (Small amount present @ 20 hours)
IODINE-125
    (Radioactivity in milk present
     for 12 days)
IODINE 131
    (Radioactivity in milk present
     for 2-14 days)
RADIOACTIVE SODIUM
    (Radioactivity in milk present
     96 hours)
TECHNETIUM-99 M
    (Radioactivity in milk present
     15 hours to 30 days)

Modified from: *Principles and Practice of Pediatrics*, Oski FA, DeAngelis CD, Feigin RD, Warshaw JB (eds), J.B. Lippincott, Philadelphia, 1990, p.546.

The Breast and The Physiology of Lactation, Creasy RK, Resnik R (eds), W.B. Saunders Company, Philadelphia, 1989, p.166.

DRUGS THAT ARE CONTRAINDICATED FOR BREAST FEEDING MOTHERS

AMETHOPTERIN
AMIODARONE
BROMIDE
BROMOCRIPTINE
CIMETIDINE*
CLEMOSTINES
CYCLOPHOSPHAMIDE
CYCLOSPORINE
DOXORUBICIN
ERGOTAMINE
GOLD SALTS
IODIDE
LITHIUM*
METHOTROXATE
METHIMAZOLE
PHENINDIONE
THIOURACIL
TIMOLOL

*   See page 302.

Modified from: *Principles and Practice of Pediatrics*, Oski FA, DeAngelis CD, Feigin RD, Warshaw JB (eds), J.B. Lippincott, Philadelphia, 1990, p.546.

CEASE BREAST FEEDING UNTIL DRUG EXCRETED

CHLORAMPHENICOL +
CLINDAMYCIN +
CLONIDINE
RADIOPHARMACEUTICALS
METRONIDAZOLE
ZOMEPIRAC +

+   See page 302.

Modified from: *The Breast and The Physiology of Lactation*, Creasy RK, Resnik R (eds), W.B. Saunders Company, Philadelphia, 1989, p.166.

USUALLY COMPATIBLE BUT ADVERSE EFFECTS REPORTED OR POSSIBLE

ANESTHETICS, SEDATIVES (AS SINGLE DOSES
  AVOID CHRONIC USE)
    Alcohol
    Chloral hydrate
    Methyprylon
    Diazepam
    Flurazepam

ANTIEPILEPTICS (AVOID CHRONIC USE, IF
  POSSIBLE)
    Carbamazepine
    Ethosuximide
    Phenobarbital
    Phenytoin
    Primidone
    Thiopental
    Valproic acid

ANTIHISTAMINES, DECONGESTANTS
    Chlorpheniramine
    Cyproheptadine
    Dexbrompheniramine maleate
      with d-isoephedrine
    Diphenhydramine
    Brompheniramine
    Ephedrine
    Pseudoephedrine

ANTIHYPERTENSIVES, CARDIOVASCULAR DRUGS
    Quinidine
    Reserpine

ANTI-INFECTIVE DRUGS
    Amantadine
    Ethambutol +
    Isoniazid +
    Methenamine
    Sulfas (avoid in immediate newborn
      period)

+   See page 302

ANTITHYROID DRUGS
    Carbimazole
    Methimazole
    Propylthiouracil
BRONCHODILATORS
    Albuterol
    Isoproterenol
    Metaproterenol
    Terbutaline
    Prednisone (in short term use)
    Theophylline
DIURETICS (MAY SUPPRESS LACTATION)
    Bendroflumethiazide
    Chlorothiazide
    Chlorthalidone
    Furosemide
    Hydrochlorothiazide
    Methyclothiazide
    Spironolactone
HORMONES
    Estrogen/progesterone contraceptive
MUSCLE RELAXANTS
    Carisoprodol
PAIN RELIEVERS
    Indomethacin
    Salicylates +
PSYCHOTROPIC AGENTS
    Antianxiety drugs
            Chlordiazepoxide
            Clorazepate
            Diazepam *
            Hydroxyzine
            Meprobamate *
            Oxazepam
            Prazepam *

*   See page 302.

Modified from: *Principles and Practice of
Pediatrics*, Oski FA, DeAngelis CD, Feigin RD, Warshaw
JB (eds), J.B. Lippincott, Philadelphia, 1990, p.546.

The Breast and The Physiology of Lactation, Creasy
RK, Resnik R (eds), W.B. Saunders Company,
Philadelphia, 1989, p.166.

BREAST FEEDING NEED NOT BE INTERRUPTED

ANESTHETICS, SEDATIVES
    Barbiturate
    Chloroform
    Diphenhydramine
    Halothane
    Hydroxyzine
    Magnesium sulfate
    Secobarbital
ANTICOAGULANTS
    Bishydroxycoumarin
    Coumadin
    Heparin
ANTIHISTAMINES, DECONGESTANTS AND
  BRONCHODILATORS
    Diphenhydramine
    Diphylline *
    Trimeprazine
    Tripelennamine
ANTIHYPERTENSIVES, CARDIOVASCULAR DRUGS
    Atenolol
    Captopril
    Digoxin
    Disopyramide
    Guanethidine
    Hydralazine
    Methyldopa
    Metoprolol *
    Nadolol *
    Propranolol
ANTI-INFECTIVE DRUGS
    Cefadroxil
    Cefazolin
    Cefotaxime
    Cephalexin
    Cepholothin
    Chloroquine
    Dicloxacillin
    Erythromycin
    Gentamicin
    Nafcillin
    Nalidixic acid
    Nitrofurantoin
    Oxacillin
    Penicillin
    Tetracycline +
    Trimethoprin
    Vancomycin

MUSCLE RELAXANTS
   Baclofen
   Methocarbamol
PAIN RELIEVERS
   Acetaminophen
   Butorphanol
   Codeine
   Flufenamic acid
   Ibuprofen
   Mefenamid acid
   Meperidine
   Methadine
   Morphine
   Naproxyn
   Oxycodone
   Phenylbutazone
   Propoxyphene
PSYCHOTROPIC AGENTS
   Antidepressants
      Amitriptyline
      Amoxapine
      Desipramine
      Dothiepin
      Imipramine
      Nortriptyline
      Tranylcypromine
   Antipsychotic drugs
      Chlorpromazine
      Haloperidol
      Mesoridazine
      Piperacetazine
      Prochlorperazine
      Thioridazine
      Trifluoperazine

   *   Accumulates in breast milk
   +   Some consider contraindicated;
         others do not. Refer to original
         sources.

Modified from: *Principles and Practice of
Pediatrics*, Oski FA, DeAngelis CD, Feigin RD, Warshaw
JB (eds), J.B. Lippincott, Philadelphia, 1990, p.546.

The Breast and The Physiology of Lactation, Creasy
RK, Resnik R (eds), W.B. Saunders Company,
Philadelphia, 1989, p.166.

DRUGS OF ABUSE THAT ARE CONTRAINDICATED IN BREAST FEEDING MOTHERS

AMPHETAMINE
COCAINE
HEROIN
MARIJUANA
NICOTINE (SMOKING)
PHENCYCLIDINE (PCP)

Modified from: *Principles and Practice of Pediatrics*, Oski FA, DeAngelis CD, Feigin RD, Warshaw JB (eds), J.B. Lippincott, Philadelphia, 1990, p.546.

The Breast and The Physiology of Lactation, Creasy RK, Resnik R (eds), W.B. Saunders Company, Philadelphia, 1989, p.166.

CHAPTER XIX

MEDICAL ORIGINS OF COMMON (AND NOT SO COMMON)
TERMS - AN ANNOTATED GLOSSARY

ALPINE SLIDE ANAPHYLAXIS

A severe allergic reaction due to contact between the skin and antigens in foliage/ground cover while alpine sliding.

AN APPLE A DAY KEEPS THE DOCTOR AWAY

This phrase has its origins in the Bible and was used by the great writer and historian of Rome, Pliny (62-113 AD). Tests carried out at Leeds University in 1981 showed fewer doctor visits by people who ate large quantities of apples compared with those who did not.

BACKPACKING NEUROPATHY

A suprascapular neuropathy resulting from prolonged backpacking.

BASEBALL FINGER

Abnormal sensation of the index finger resulting from digital ischemia.

BEER DRINKER'S CARDIOMYOPATHY

A toxin induced cardiomyopathy caused by cobalt, a defoaming agent added in the production of beer in certain parts of the world.

"BERSERK" HYPERTENSION

A form of hypertension caused by the intense excitement experienced by some playing the video game "Berserk".

BUBBLE GUM CONSTIPATION

That form of constipation resulting from swallowed chewing gum obstructing the gut.

BUFFERS BELLY

Abdominal pain resulting from pancreatic inflammation; seen largely in buffers (individuals using commercial floor polishing machines who use their belly to push or direct the handle).

CHEESE TURNERS' HYPOGLYCEMIA

A complication seen in diabetics who are "cheese turners." Cheese turners are employed to periodically rotate large blocks of aging cheese. They compress the blocks against the abdominal wall causing accelerated release of injected insulin.

CHEWING GUM HYPERAMYLASEMIA

That form of hyperamylasemia due to excessive compression and stretching of the parotid glands from rapid action of the masseter muscles while chewing gum.

CHEWING TOBACCO HYPERTENSION

That hypertension resulting from chewing tobacco which contains a substance which inhibits 11 beta-hydroxysteroid dehydrogenase.

A CLOSE SHAVE

Origins relate to the 17th century when barbers were surgeons. They practiced first by "shaving fools." Many a fool had "a close shave."

CROCODILE TEARS

Common usage refers to the hypocritical shedding of tears; term arises from the early belief that crocodiles wept while devouring their victims. Indeed, this is correct but only because opening and closing of the jaws in crocodiles causes the tear ducts to discharge automatically.

DOPE

One meaning refers to a request for a soda fountain order ("gimme a dope"), circa 1865 to 1886 when Coca-Cola was real Coke since it contained cocaine, subsequently replaced by caffeine.

FLUTIST NEUROPATHY

A form of pressure neuropathy caused by playing the flute. The first common digital nerve is affected.

GOOSE STEP HEMATURIA

That form of hematuria associated with "power walking" (also loosely called "goose stepping").

GRECIAN FORMULA PLUMBISM

A little known cause of lead poisoning following the ingestion instead of topical application of Grecian Formula, a hair darkening agent whose active ingredient is a lead salt.

HIS NAME IS MUD

Mud refers to Dr. Samuel Mudd, the unfortunate physician chosen by John Wilkes Booth to set his leg. Mudd, sentenced to life for conspiracy, was a man whose name began the term "mud."

HOLY COMMUNION DIARRHEA

A well described form of diarrhea observed in subjects with celiac disease who partake of communion which is prepared from unleavened wheat flour.

HUFFY BIKE HEMATURIA

A form of gross or microscopic hematuria seen in boys who bounce about on dirt bicycles. Anatomical source of the hematuria is speculative.

HYDROX FECALIS

A condition characterized by black stools and reported to be due to the excessive consumption of Oreo cookies.

JAZZ DANCER'S BOTTOM

A condition resulting from excessive
compression of the gluteal area during
"bottoms down" while performing jazz
dancing maneuvers. May result in
sciatica.

JOGGER'S LEUKOCYTOSIS

That form of leukocytosis resulting from
the perversion jogging. A 10,000 M run
results in a 50% rise in the white blood
cell count.

KICK THE BUCKET

To die; not referring to the vessel used
for carrying water, but to the bucket
beam, or wooden frame on which pigs were
hung after slaughter; therefore, anyone
who has died may have "kicked the
bucket."

KOOL-AID COLITIS

A guaiac negative red stool resulting
from ingestion of Kool Aid.

LASER PRINTER RHINITIS

Irritation of the nasal mucosa from
inhalation of volatile hydrocarbons,
combustion products of styrene -
butadine toners.

LONG IN THE TOOTH

Getting on in years. Does not mean that the teeth continue to grow in humans but rather refers to horses who, as they age, have receding gum lines giving the appearance of looking "long in the tooth."

MAD AS A HATTER

Origin reflects the mental condition of hatters who years ago used mercury (and were poisoned by it) in the treatment of furs to make felt.

MARATHON RUNNER'S STOOL

A guaiac positive stool, an almost invariable finding after a full marathon.

MORTICIAN'S GYNECOMASTIA

Enlargement of the breasts seen in undertakers (presumably male), due to the absorption through the skin of bare hands of estrogen-like substances in formaldehyde solutions.

NERDS TURDS

A grossly bloody/pinkish appearance of the stool following the ingestion of large quantities of the cereal "Nerds."

NINE-BALL NECK

A soreness of the neck and trapezius areas resulting from prolonged bending over while playing billiards.

NINTENDINITIS

A form of tendinitis of the thumb or forefinger resulting from frequent repetitive depression of the hand controls of Nintendo.

PAC MAN THUMB

Intense pain on movement of the thumb from repetitive or sustained action of the thumb on the controls of Pac Man videos.

PEDAL PUSHER'S PALSY

A sciatic nerve palsy from excessive exercise bicycle usage.

PISS

Origin unknown, but thought to be derived from the sound of the activity (echoic).

POTTER'S FIELD

A burial ground for the unidentified or unclaimed dead. Origin is in Matthew 27:7 which recounts how the rejected thirty pieces of Judas' silver was used to buy, as a burial place for the poor, a field that belonged to a potter.

ST. VITUS DANCE

An uncommon synonym for the chorea of rheumatic fever. Chorea mimics the wild form of dancing used to celebrate the feast day of the Christian martyr during Medieval times.

SCUT BOOK

A daybook in earlier (or not so earlier) times in which senior doctors list "dirty work" for interns such as stool tests. Scut is derived from the rootword "shit", meaning to make a mess of.

SIGN OF THE CHESHIRE CAT

A facies characterized by a peculiarly rigid smile in the shape of the cheshire cat. Seen in some subjects with neurologic disorders characterized by dystonia.

SPACE INVADER'S EPILEPSY

A photic induced seizure in individuals with an underlying seizure disorder, induced by even transient playing of Space Invaders.

SUNFLOWER SEED CONSTIPATION

That form of constipation resulting from obstruction of the gut in association with massive sunflower seed ingestion.

SWIMMING GOGGLE NEUROPATHY

> A neuropathy characterized by loss of sensation along the supraorbital (V-1) nerve.

SWIMMING POOL GIARDIASIS

> That form of diarrhea resulting from swimming with the "fishes" (Polymastigida) in improperly chlorinated community swimming pools.

TEA DRINKER'S ANEMIA

> That anemia presumably due to iron deficiency resulting from the binding of iron to tannin containing beverages. This results in a failure to absorb iron from the diet.

TYPHOID MARY DIARRHEA

> That form of diarrhea caused by certain strains of salmonella. Origin: Mary Mallon, an immigrant cook in 1888.

VIDEO **ANGINA**

A disorder noted mostly in adults characterized by true angina after prolonged viewing of CRT screens. An occupational hazard.

VIDEO **CAMERA AMBLYOPIA**

A disorder characterized by transient blindness in one eye resulting from prolonged view finder use of modern day home video cameras.

X-RAY

"X" refers to any unknown. The ray producing the film image was unknown and simply called "X".

Index

A

H

N